Prostate Disease

Prostate Disease

The Most Comprehensive,
Up-to-Date Information Available
to Help You Understand Your Condition,
Make the Right Treatment Choices,
and Cope Effectively

W. Scott McDougal, M.D., with P. J. Skerrett

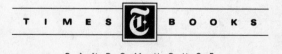

TIMES 𝕿 BOOKS

RANDOM HOUSE

This book cannot and must not replace hands-on medical care or the specific advice of your doctor. Use it instead to help you ask the right questions, make the right choices, and work more closely with your doctor and other members of your health-care team.

Library of Congress Cataloging-in-Publication Data

McDougal, W. Scott (William Scott)
   Prostate Disease: the most comprehensive, up-to-date information available to help you understand your condition, make the right treatment choices, and cope effectively / W. Scott McDougal, with P.J. Skerrett.—1st ed.
      p.   cm.
   Includes index.
   ISBN 0-8129-2319-7
   1. Prostate—Cancer—Popular works.   2. Prostate—Diseases—Popular works.   I. Skerrett, P. J. (Patrick J.), 1953–   .
II. Title.
RC280.P7M33   1995
616.6'5—dc20   95-15175

Designed by Levavi & Levavi
Manufactured in the United States of America

9 8 7 6 5 4 3 2

Acknowledgments

Several years ago, the staff of Massachusetts General Hospital set out to create a series of medical guides that would help all patients become more effective partners in their health care. We wanted to create clearly written, authoritative books that reflected a number of voices critical to the health care team, including doctors, nurses, dietitians, social workers, therapists, and, of course, the patients themselves. We are pleased that with this book the series has become a reality.

We wish to thank John Taylor Williams and the Palmer & Dodge Agency for first suggesting the idea for this series. Martin S. Bander, then the hospital's director of news and public affairs and deputy to the hospital's CEO, has been an invaluable editor and coordinator for the series; we are indebted to him for his advice and guiding hand. We wish to further thank Richard Kitz, M.D., of Massachusetts General Hospital, who heads the series committee of physicians and allied health professionals who have made these books possible.

We also wish to thank the staff of Times Books, in particular publisher Peter Osnos and executive editor Elizabeth Rapoport, for their editorial guidance and publishing support.

Many other people made other substantial contributions that clearly enriched this book. We would especially like to thank the dozens of men who shared their stories about fighting prostate cancer, or dealing with BPH or prostatitis. We hope that what they learned about making decisions or coping will make it easier for others.

Dr. William U. Shipley, Radiation Oncology, and Dr. Donald S. Kaufman, Hematology/Oncology, made major contributions to the chapters for which they acted as coauthors. The nurses of Bigelow 11, especially head nurse Mary McDonough, offered helpful pointers gleaned from their work with men hospitalized for a prostate problem or recovering from prostate surgery. MGH physicians Alex Althausen, Elizabeth Bailey, Michael Barry, David Borsook, Frank McGovern, Niall Heney, and Anthony Zeitman shared their expertise, as did nurses William Casey, Katie Mannix, and Elizabeth Montgomery. Three clinicians from the Dana-Farber Cancer Institute in Boston, psychiatrist Patricia Perri Rieker and physicians James Talcott and Kerry Kilbridge, contributed important data on coping with prostate cancer.

The best insights and advice in the pages that follow often belong to those mentioned above; any errors or omissions are ours.

Contents

Introduction

Even in this era of heightened health awareness, prostate disease remains an essentially private, almost taboo topic. That's too bad, since the majority of American men will be touched by prostate disease at some time in their lives. Some will suffer a single episode of infection—bacterial prostatitis—that disappears forever after treatment with antibiotics. The majority, however, will deal with prostate problems for years. And almost as many men die of prostate cancer each year as women die from breast cancer.

There are three categories of prostate trouble: *prostatitis,* an inflammation of the gland; *benign prostatic hyperplasia,* or BPH, a noncancerous enlargement of the prostate that usually begins in middle age; and *prostate cancer.* To give you an idea of their impact, here are some numbers: prostatitis accounts for almost 2 million physician visits a year; more than half of all men over age 60 have BPH; and approximately a quarter of a million men will be diagnosed with prostate cancer this year alone.

Prostatitis, BPH, and prostate cancer have different health risks. The first two are irritating rather than life threatening, while prostate cancer kills more than 40,000 men each year. But because they all afflict the same lime-sized gland, they share similar symptoms and side effects. Since the prostate sits right where the urinary and reproductive systems merge, most of these have to do with urination or sex, and can dramatically alter the quality of a man's life.

Even though physicians have been diagnosing and treating prostate problems for millennia—flexible catheters used to drain urine from men with enlarged prostates were found preserved in the rubble of Pompeii—there is still an awful lot we don't know about them. We don't know, for example, exactly what physical or chemical signal makes the prostate begin enlarging in virtually all older men. Nor do we know what causes prostate cancer. And there is considerable debate about the best ways to treat prostatitis, BPH, and prostate cancer. Important advances are made nearly every month, but we still have much to learn.

This uncertainty about causes and treatments, plus the long-term nature of prostate diseases and their potential for life-changing complications, mean that men are often forced to make some exceedingly difficult decisions. Say you've just been diagnosed with benign prostatic hyperplasia. Your physician tells you it can be treated with drugs, surgery, or a no-treatment approach called watchful waiting, and then leaves the ultimate decision up to you. Why? Because only you can decide if you want to risk the slight risks associated with surgery, or live with the potential side effects of drug therapy, or merely watch and wait and see what happens over the next few months.

In other words, you are going to have to learn as much as you can about prostate disease in order to make wise, informed decisions about your treatment. Reading this book is a good start. Talking with men who have already faced these issues can be equally helpful. The national support groups listed in the Resources chapter can point you to a local support group and men in your area who can offer valuable, personal perspectives.

One final thought before we get underway. Because most prostate problems are slow to develop, you have plenty of time to make a careful, well-informed decision about treatment. Prostate cancer and BPH develop over years—early-stage prostate cancer is generally one of the slowest growing cancers known—so taking a few weeks to learn about your options and discuss them with your physician or members of a support group won't endanger your life. In fact, such a deliberate approach will help you come to a decision that is not only medically sound but feels right. And that, in the long run, is a crucial component of treatment and recovery.

Prostate Disease

1

The Prostate

Given the ills and anguish the prostate causes millions of men each year, you'd expect it to be a large, impressive gland. That's not the case. It's half the size of an egg in a young man, and a man can easily live a long and healthy life without one. The old adage about the three most important things in real estate—location, location, and location—applies neatly to the prostate. It wields tremendous influence over men's lives because it sits at the physiological intersection of urination and sex. The prostate wraps around the urethra, the tube that carries urine from bladder to penis. The same tube also transports semen from several reproductive glands to the penis. So prostate problems usually lead to difficulty urinating or they may disrupt fertility or sexual activity.

Functions

A baby boy is born with a pea-sized prostate gland. Over the next ten to twelve years, the prostate grows only a little. Then, with the onset of puberty, the gland begins a stage of explosive growth that lasts several years. By the late teens or early twenties, the average man's prostate measures about the size of a golf ball and weighs about three-fourths of an ounce (fig. 1.1).

It's no coincidence that this growth spurt comes during the period of sexual maturation. The gland's main function in life is manufacturing and secreting substances that accompany sperm cells on their reproductive journey. Several prostate-made buffers neutralize acidic vaginal secretions that can kill unprotected sperm. The prostate adds prostaglandins to semen to help relax the cervix, allowing sperm cells entry to the uterus. And fructose, a sugar produced by the seminal vesicles attached to the prostate, provides sperm with a perfect source of energy to power

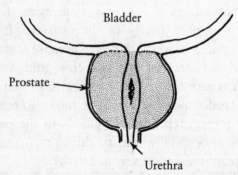

Figure 1.1. *In a young man, the prostate gland is about the size of a lime. It surrounds the urethra, the tube that carries urine from the bladder to the penis.*

them on their long swim through the female reproductive system.

The prostate is really a collection of thirty to fifty tiny glands, each emptying into small ducts that lead to the urethra. During an orgasm, muscles in and around the prostate contract, squeezing the glands' secretions into the urethra. There they blend with sperm cells propelled upward from the testes and with fluids from the seminal vesicles. The entire mixture is called semen. Wavelike contractions of the urethra push semen down the tube and out the penis in spurts.

The prostate may have another function—protecting the reproductive tract from infection. The gland is strategically placed below the bladder and beneath the openings to critical components of the reproductive system. Bacteria and other microbes can easily work their way into the penis's opening and inch their way through the urethra and into the seminal vesicles or testes. Secretions from the prostate help prevent microbes from making this trek. In some men, however, this process backfires and the prostate itself becomes the source of chronic infections (see Chapter 2).

The gland sits at a strategic spot for all of its functions (fig. 1.2). It nestles just below the bladder and surrounds the urethra. In fact, the prostate gland and urethra are so intimately connected that in order to remove the gland, a surgeon must sever the urethra above and below the prostate, then sew the cut ends together, re-creating an unbroken tube. You can picture the prostate as a small apple standing stem-end up. The skin represents the prostate's tough, muscular coat, or capsule. The pulp represents the gland itself, and the core the urethra. Just as with core and pulp, urethra and prostate grow into each

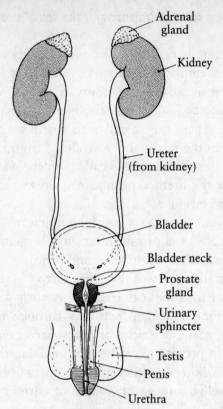

Figure 1.2. *The male genitourinary system is made up of several interconnected parts. The kidneys produce urine, which trickles through the ureters to the bladder, an elastic storage pouch. At voiding, the bladder contracts, propelling urine through the urethra and out the penis. The testes manufacture sperm. During orgasm, sperm are pumped up to the prostate, where they mix with secretions from the seminal vesicles and prostate. This fluid, called semen, enters the urethra inside the prostate and is then ejaculated.*

other, making it impossible to tell where one begins and the other ends.

For normal daily function, this arrangement works

beautifully. The prostate can dump its contents directly into the urethra, which also acts as the male reproductive channel. At the critical moment of ejaculation, muscles in and around the upper end of the prostate and the bladder neck squeeze secretions from the prostate, testes, and seminal vesicles through the urethra.

Prostate trouble may disrupt the gland's normal functions. A swollen or chronically infected prostate can stop manufacturing critical components of semen, decreasing a man's fertility. Or it can make ejaculation painful. Just as likely, a swollen or tumor-bearing gland makes urination difficult. When the gland enlarges due to infection, benign growth, or a tumor, the tough outer coat restricts any outward expansion. Instead, the pent-up growth is directed inward toward the flexible urethra, squeezing and narrowing this tube. And that spells trouble.

Think of it this way: Imagine you're trying to drain a flooded basement with a fire hose and a diesel pump. Halfway through, the fire department shows up to reclaim its hose and you have to switch to a standard garden hose. Now the job will take longer, and the pump will have to work harder. The same relationship exists between the bladder and the urethra. If the tube narrows, urine won't flow out as freely. And this can start a chain reaction that involves the bladder, leading to a variety of urinary problems ranging from the need to urinate several times a night to a sudden inability to urinate at all.

Underneath its fibrous coat, the prostate is organized into four distinct regions or zones. The *peripheral zone* abuts the rectum and makes up 75 percent of the prostate. Most cancers arise here. The *central zone* is almost pure secretory gland, and makes up about 20 percent of the prostate. The tiny zone of *preprostatic tissue* wraps around the urethra where it emerges from the bladder. During ejaculation it contracts tightly, preventing semen from being pushed backward into the bladder. Finally, the *transition zone* normally occupies a small area immediately around the urethra, making up about 5 percent of prostate volume in a young man. But this tissue begins growing late in life. It quadruples or octuples in size, compressing the urethra and giving rise to benign prostatic hyperplasia, the scourge of millions of middle-aged and elderly men.

It would be less than accurate to think of the prostate as hanging suspended from the flexible urethra, bobbing around every time you move. Ligaments anchor the prostate, and thus the urethra, to the pubic bone. And the gland is actually embedded in tissue, which further holds it in place (fig. 1.3). Sheets of tissue also attach it to the

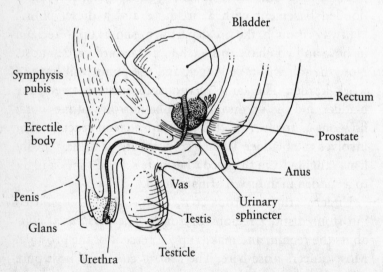

Figure 1.3. *The prostate sits right next to the rectum, making it relatively easy for a physician to check its condition.*

bladder. Finally, it rests atop the rectum. That's a good thing, since this connection allows a physician to check the prostate's health by feeling it through the rectum. This technique, called the digital rectal exam, is a mainstay for detecting cancer and other prostate ills.

Like every other organ, gland, or tissue, the prostate gets its nourishment from a network of arteries and rids itself of wastes via small veins and lymph vessels. The latter collect lymph, a milky fluid containing white blood cells, proteins, and other substances that accumulate in the spaces between cells. Enlargements called nodes appear every so often along the network of lymphatic vessels. White blood cells inside these nodes break down cell debris and attack bacteria, wayward cells, or other foreign particles. Like veins, lymph vessels gradually merge into larger and larger tubes, and finally dump their lymphatic fluid into the heart where it mixes with blood.

Nerves running into the prostate control contractions during orgasm as well as other as-yet-undiscovered functions. For years, urologists (physicians specializing in urinary disorders and male reproductive problems) believed that the nerves controlling erections ran from the spinal cord through the prostate and down into the penis. In the late 1970s, two physicians discovered that these nerves actually run along the outer coat, essentially using the gland for support.

Structure

Most men are never really aware that they have a prostate gland until late middle age. It usually works smoothly and unobtrusively, another small organ that's generally taken for granted. But when it malfunctions, from an infection or excessive growth, it causes tremendous inconvenience.

The following chapters describe the ailments that befall this small gland, and how they can be treated.

2

Inflammation of the Prostate (Prostatitis)

Inflamed, infected, and irritated prostates cause pain and anguish among men of all ages. Some immediately worry that prostate pain means cancer and delay going to the doctor because they've heard that treatment for prostate cancer makes a man impotent. Others try to ignore the problem, hoping it will disappear on its own. Many men are too embarrassed to talk with friends or a physician about "private" pains or trouble urinating. Odds are, though, that a coworker, golfing partner, or church acquaintance is suffering the same way. Infected or inflamed prostates account for an estimated 2 million visits to the doctor each year. Unlike other prostate problems, this one afflicts young men as well as older men.

What It Is

Prostatitis is a catchall term covering a range of prostate problems. Physicians traditionally talk about four sepa-

rate categories—acute bacterial prostatitis, chronic bacterial prostatitis, nonbacterial prostatitis, and prostatodynia—though all four come with similar symptoms. These
include a burning sensation deep inside the penis; pain
when urinating; frequent or urgent urination, sometimes
accompanied by dribbling; discomfort during and after
ejaculation; and lower back pain or pain in the entire genital region. Prostatitis can strike a man just once in his lifetime and disappear after treatment. Or it can linger for
months, even years, and reappear regularly.

Although prostate cancer dominates the news, don't immediately assume that sudden trouble urinating or a
brand-new pain inside the penis heralds the sudden onset
of a tumor. Actually, it's more likely prostatitis, since tumors tend to grow rather slowly and symptoms appear
more gradually. But just to make sure, your physician will
invariably check for suspicious lumps or bumps to rule
out cancer as a possible cause of symptoms. This can be
accomplished with two of the quick, simple tests described
below.

A single bout of prostatitis is no more harmful than a
case of the flu or a sinus infection. But don't take this ailment for granted. Unchecked, untreated prostatitis can
evolve into chronic disease. Not only is this problem difficult to eradicate and frustrating to live with, but it can
make you less fertile and interfere with your ability to father a child.

Diagnostic Tests

As the name implies, bacterial prostatitis arises from infection with a bacterium or other microbe. In some cases it
results from an overactive or faulty immune system that

attacks normal, healthy prostate tissue. (A haywire immune system is thought to cause a variety of ills, ranging from arthritis to psoriasis and lupus.) And some prostatitis appears as a physiological symptom of stress. Telling one kind from another, and all of them from prostate cancer, requires a few of these basic tests:

MEDICAL HISTORY

The taking of your medical history is one of the most crucial parts of a visit to any physician. Sometimes just telling your urologist, internist, or family physician everything you can about the problem is enough to prompt an accurate diagnosis. Try to describe as specifically as you can where and when it hurts, when the trouble began, your urinary and sexual habits, other ailments you might have, any medications you might be taking, and anything else that might be pertinent.

DIGITAL (FINGER) RECTAL EXAM

By simply feeling the prostate gland, a physician can tell a lot about its condition (fig. 2.1). You'll lie on your side on an examining table, feet drawn up, or stand and bend over a table, as your physician inserts a gloved, well-lubricated finger into your rectum and gently presses the adjoining prostate. Some men find this procedure uncomfortable or embarrassing. Relax, think of something pleasant, and it will be over in a few seconds. A normal gland feels firm but pliable, much like the tip of your nose or the pad of your hand. An infected gland may feel swollen or mushy, what urologists call "boggy." A small, hard lump or nodule could indicate cancer, and its presence generally leads to a biopsy and other tests (see Chapter 6).

Rectal Exam

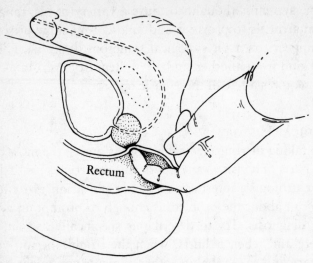

Rectum

Figure 2.1. *Using the tip of a finger, a physician can digitally inspect the surface of the prostate, looking for any suspicious bumps or changes in texture.*

PSA Test

In tandem with a rectal exam, your physician will draw a small sample of blood from your arm and test it for prostate-specific antigen, or PSA. This is a protein that rarely gets into the bloodstream in large amounts unless something such as an infection, excess growth, or cancer forces it there. Men with normal-sized prostates have anywhere from zero to 4.0 nanograms of PSA per milliliter of blood. (That's four-millionths of a gram per liter.) Levels above 4.0, however, suggest that something is awry, either an infection, benign growth, or a tumor. An above-normal PSA will almost invariably compel your physician to do other tests if there's any question about the diagnosis.

URINALYSIS

This involves nothing more than washing your hands, cleaning the head of your penis with an antiseptic wipe, and urinating into a sterile plastic cup. In the laboratory, a technician examines your urine sample under the microscope for bacteria, white blood cells, or sediment. All of these suggest an active infection. In order to determine the kind of bacteria present and their sensitivity to specific antibiotics, a few drops of urine may be spread on glass plates coated with nutrients that encourage bacterial growth.

PROSTATE MASSAGE

This somewhat-less-than-pleasant test allows your physician to find an infection or inflammation in the prostate that hasn't spilled over into the bladder or urethra. Starting with a full bladder, you'll void a few ounces of urine into one cup, then another, and then stop urinating before your bladder is empty. Next you'll lean over a table and tightly hold the tip of your penis to prevent any fluid from leaking out. Your physician will insert a gloved finger into your rectum and press down on the prostate several times, forcing its stored fluid into the urethra. During this procedure you'll feel as though you desperately need to urinate. Once the massage is over, you'll immediately urinate into a third cup, and then finally empty your bladder into the toilet. The third sample, rich in prostate fluids, will be examined under a microscope for telltale signs of infection. These include the microbes themselves, or white blood cells called leukocytes, which nearly always migrate to the site of an infection.

URODYNAMIC TESTS

When there's no obvious cause like bacteria or white blood cells for prostate pain or irritation, your physician may take a look at how your bladder, urethra, and other associated muscles work together during urination. The simplest test involves voiding into a specially equipped toilet that measures the rate of urine flow (how many milliliters of fluid per second). Or your doctor may place a catheter inside your bladder that measures the amount of pressure exerted during urination and the amount of urine left in the bladder once you've finished.

Difficulties of Treatment

It can take some men months or years (or never) to rid themselves of prostatitis. Why this difficulty? One hurdle is the gland's physiology. The fluids it makes are for use outside the body, not inside. So the gland is covered with a thick capsule that doesn't allow these fluids to cross over into the bloodstream. That also means it's difficult for substances dissolved in the blood, like antibiotics, to get into prostate tissue. The other reason that prostatitis can be so difficult to treat is that we can't always find exactly what's causing the problem.

Types of Prostatitis and Treatments

Acute Bacterial Prostatitis

Acute bacterial prostatitis hits mostly young to middle-aged men. It often strikes suddenly. For an otherwise healthy man, the symptoms of acute bacterial prostatitis can be frightening. They often start with a high fever, accompanied by a burning deep inside the penis, especially during urination. Testicular and back pain are common, as is discomfort during and after ejaculation. The normal pattern and rhythm of urination are also thrown off kilter. That means getting up at night to urinate, or having to urinate with greater urgency, or dribbling instead of producing a strong stream.

The prostate, like virtually every other organ, gland, or tissue in the body, can be colonized by bacteria, fungi, viruses, or other strange organisms. The main route into the prostate is through the penis. Bacteria can migrate from the opening of the penis into the urethra, prostate, and other tissues. This often happens as a result of sexual activity, making prostatitis an often-overlooked symptom of sexually transmitted disease. Bacteria or other microbes can also get deposited in the prostate when urine accidentally backs up into the gland on its way from bladder to penis. No matter how foreign organisms get there, under the right conditions they can make themselves comfortable and flourish.

Diagnosing acute bacterial prostatitis doesn't generally present a big challenge. A man's description of his symptoms will often lead a physician directly to the culprit. Next comes a rectal exam, partly to rule out cancer and partly to check the prostate's condition. In acute bacterial prostatitis, the gland is tender and swollen with infection-fighting white blood cells and fluids. The key diagnostic tool is the urine test. If a sample of freshly voided urine is packed with bacteria and white blood cells, then acute bacterial prostatitis is most likely the cause of the trouble.

Treatment depends on how sick the infection has made its victim. An extremely high fever, dehydration, or the inability to urinate sometimes require a trip to the hospital.

There, intravenous antibiotics and fluids can be administered. Or, if the infection has swollen the prostate so it squeezes the urethra shut, a catheter to drain away urine can be threaded through the abdomen directly into the bladder. Normally, once the antibiotics kick in and start decimating the infection, the ability to urinate quickly returns.

You may need bed rest until the fever has dropped, taking antibiotics specifically prescribed for this ailment and drinking plenty of fluids to frequently flush the bladder and urethra. Anti-inflammatory drugs such as ibuprofen can help ease the pain.

For unknown reasons, drugs don't get into the prostate gland as easily as they do the kidney or lungs. So antibiotic therapy often lasts for a month, just to make sure that enough of the drug reaches its target. One of the greatest mistakes men with acute bacterial prostatitis make is failing to finish the entire prescribed course of drugs. Stopping too soon spares bacteria living in protected little pockets. They can either flare up into another full-blown infection or develop resistance to the antibiotics. This scenario may convert a single case of potentially curable acute bacterial prostatitis into chronic bacterial prostatitis. So make sure you follow your physician's recommendation and take the antibiotics for the full term prescribed, even if your symptoms disappear within a few days.

Chronic Bacterial Prostatitis

More common in older than younger men, chronic bacterial prostatitis can be a frustrating, irritating problem that lasts for months or years. It shares many symptoms with its acute sibling, though the chronic infections tend to be less dramatic. It may or may not come with painful urination, an inability to urinate, the urge to urinate frequently, tenderness between the rectum and scrotum, or pain during or after ejaculation. The hallmark of this condition is recurrent urinary tract infections.

A prostate massage, described earlier, helps tell chronic bacterial prostatitis from nonbacterial prostatitis. In general, both have negative urine cultures, meaning no microbes show up in the urine. But one sign of chronic bacterial prostatitis is prostate fluid rich in bacteria or white blood cells.

No one knows why antibiotic treatment doesn't permanently rid all men of their prostate infections. In some cases, bacteria are traded back and forth during sexual activity between a monogamous couple, causing recurrent infections in both parties. Men who don't use condoms and have more than one sexual partner can continually pick up microbes that infect the urethra or prostate. Prostate stones may also play a role. About three-quarters of middle-aged men and all elderly men accumulate tiny, insoluble crystals deep inside the gland. They're usually made of compounds found only in urine. Some researchers believe the stones form when urine leaks into the prostate despite the one-way valves meant to release prostate fluids into the urethra while keeping urine, sperm, and seminal fluid out. These "prostatic calculi" may act as hiding places for bacteria or other microbes and protect them from being destroyed by white blood cells or killed by antibiotics.

Basic treatment for chronic bacterial prostatitis involves bacteria-killing drugs. Because the infection may be extraordinarily hard to eradicate, standard therapy starts with twelve to sixteen weeks of daily antibiotics. It's crucial to follow the program for the entire time, even if the infection appears to be under control—it may just be hiding deep in the prostate or inside some stones. While this is the best therapy yet devised, it banishes chronic bacterial prostatitis in only 30 to 40 percent of men.

Another, more radical approach that provides relief for some men is a surgical procedure called transurethral resection of the prostate, or TURP. This operation is performed through the urethra, and removes virtually all of the stone-filled prostate. However, there's little information available to suggest that this procedure works any better than drug therapy. And since it requires anesthesia, a hospital stay, and may cause abnormal ejaculations (and subsequent infertility), you don't want to pick this option without careful consideration. (See Chapter 3 for a description of the TURP and its side effects.)

Nonbacterial Prostatitis

Another prostate problem for which there is no easy solution is nonbacterial prostatitis. It is by far the most common of all the prostate-irritating diseases, accounting for roughly two-thirds of all cases. It differs from the preceding two in a small but significant way: the prostate gets inflamed but no bacteria can be found in the urine or prostate fluids. Other than that, it shares symptoms with its cousins—frequent urination, especially at night; a weak or interrupted urine stream, sometimes with dribbling at the end; postejaculatory pain; or general pain in the genital region. It also tends to persist. Paul, a forty-six-year-old oil company executive, has lived with nonbacterial prostatitis for more than ten years. It started out of the blue. "While driving to work one day I got this strange pain. Now I've adapted much of my life around it. I sit on a special cushion because hard chairs give me a pain. I always take an aisle seat in airplanes so I don't have to keep climbing over people to get to the bathroom. And ejaculations aren't as much fun anymore, since they usually come with a deep pain."

Exactly what causes nonbacterial prostatitis (and prostatodynia, described below) remains a mystery. A healthy prostate makes about one-tenth of a teaspoon of fluid a day; five times that when its owner is sexually aroused. This prostatic fluid is ejaculated out of the body or, if a man is not sexually active, either leaked into the urine or continually absorbed and recycled. A sudden, dramatic increase in sexual activity can make the prostate work overtime and cause some irritation or pain. The opposite is also true. If a man who is used to ejaculating once or twice a day suddenly stops for a period, his pumped-up prostate can become congested with excess fluid that has nowhere to go.

Some researchers think the culprit may be a microbe called chlamydia, a tricky organism larger than a virus but smaller than a bacterium. In men and women alike it causes the most common sexually transmitted disease in the United States, nonspecific urethritis. Men infected with chlamydia often see a clear or pus-filled fluid oozing from the tip of the penis, or find a drop of fluid on their shorts. Many feel some burning or pain when they urinate. Chlamydia may migrate along the urethra and into the prostate, prompting a nonbacterial infection and inflammatory response. Other researchers point to mycoplasmas, the smallest free-living organisms known, as a possible cause of nonbacterial prostatitis. Fungi and viruses have also been implicated. Or perhaps the cause isn't an organism. Urine leaking into the prostate can irritate the gland and set off an inflammatory response much like that induced by an infection. Nonbacterial prostatitis could also be caused by an autoimmune disease like diabetes, lupus, or arthritis in which the body unwittingly identifies "self" proteins as foreign and attacks them. Perhaps there's no single cause, and a variety of different diseases all lead to similar symptoms that we call prostatitis.

Without an identifiable cause, treatment strategies are of the trial-and-error variety. The first line is usually drug therapy, generally a two- to four-week course of antibiotics. If that works, then the cause was probably a chlamydia-like organism. If that doesn't work, a frank discussion is in order. First and foremost, be reassured that this problem will not lead to cancer or impotence. Then realize there's no magic bullet and you may need to alter your lifestyle a bit. In some ways, living with chronic prostatitis is no different from living with other common inflammatory diseases such as arthritis and bursitis. Like them, nonbacterial prostatitis can constantly linger in the background, or flare and disappear over and over.

Controlling symptoms is the aim of most therapies for nonbacterial prostatitis. Some men find it helpful to cut down on caffeine, alcohol, or spicy foods. The first two can irritate the bladder, making urinary symptoms worse. Several compounds in cayenne pepper and other spices aren't fully broken down by the time they pass out of the kidney and can irritate the urethra on the way out. Other men can drink coffee and eat Mexican food washed down with a cold beer without feeling a twinge. Pain inside the penis or around the rectum can sometimes be alleviated with a hot sitz bath. Nonsteroidal anti-inflammatory agents such as ibuprofen often help relieve burning or pain. Some men gain relief from drugs called alpha-blockers, which relax smooth muscle inside the prostate, urethra, and bladder. And some researchers are testing a technique called transrectal hyperthermia, which heats up the prostate using the same kind of microwaves you use to boil water or cook a frozen dinner.

By far the most pleasant remedy for some prostate irritation is sexual activity. Since nonbacterial prostatitis may possibly stem from prostate congestion, regular ejaculations can keep fluids from building up inside the gland. "Regular" means whatever is regular for *you*—if you normally ejaculate once a day, then try to stick with that schedule.

Prostatodynia

Another disease with no known cause, prostatodynia affects thousands of men, most of them young to middle-aged. Like the three other types of prostatitis, it announces its presence with pain inside the penis, testicles, or groin. Voiding problems are also common—the inability to start or stop urinating, urinating in pulses, a noticeably weaker or slower stream, and increased frequency or urgency. Foreign organisms aren't thought to be responsible for this disease. Instead, it appears to come from within. Stress could account for the symptoms, as could some nerve or muscle defect that interferes with urination.

A rectal exam, urine test, and prostate massage can often rule out bacterial prostatitis as the cause of these problems. If your physician suspects prostatodynia, she or he might recommend a urodynamic test to measure urinary flow rates. Such a test can also tell if the different muscles needed for the seemingly simple (but actually quite complex) act of urination work together as they should. In some men the test reveals something called bladder-neck/urethral-spasm syndrome, characterized by sudden, uncontrollable contractions of the muscle at the base of the bladder and the smooth muscle lining the urethra as it goes through the prostate. These spasms dramatically increase the pressure inside the urethra, potentially forcing small amounts of urine backward through normally one-way ducts into the prostate. Once there, urine irritates the prostate and triggers an inflammatory response.

In other men, urodynamic testing detects spasms in the broad muscle forming the floor of the pelvis. This sling of muscle supports the abdominal organs. It's also the muscle you contract to squirt out the last drops of urine or keep yourself from passing gas. Spasms in the pelvic muscle may begin with habitual tensing in response to stress or aggravation. Eventually this unconscious action overstimulates the muscle and makes it hypersensitive, so the thinking goes, eventually escalating into uncontrollable spasms. This strain not only hurts the muscle and causes localized pain, but it may also increase pressure in the urethra and force urine up into the prostate.

A class of drugs called alpha-blockers relax the muscles around the bladder, at the bladder neck, and inside the urethra. They can neutralize smooth-muscle spasms, and lessen the pain that accompanies them. This relaxation also reduces the opportunity for urine to leak into the prostate. It may take several trial runs to find the right daily dosage of alpha-blocker.

Another possible treatment for any form of prostatitis is zinc. Some physicians encourage prostatitis sufferers to take this metallic compound, others don't. Here's the story: All tissues in the body contain very small amounts of zinc. The healthy prostate contains lots of it. Zinc keeps bacteria from entering the body. Men with prostatitis generally have below-normal zinc levels in their prostate secretions.

No one knows whether low zinc levels are the *result* of prostatitis, or whether low zinc levels *cause* prostatitis. If the former, taking zinc won't help. If the latter, it might. But then again it might not, since studies show that zinc dissolved in the blood has a hard time crossing over into prostate tissue.

If your physician suggests that you take zinc supplements, or you decide it might be a good idea, don't overdo it. Too much zinc can throw a monkey wrench into your immune system. A safe dose is fifty milligrams per day. You can also get extra zinc by eating foods rich in this mineral. These include pumpkin seeds, lentils, oysters, wheat germ, bran, eggs, and peas.

3

Benign Prostatic Hyperplasia (Enlarged Prostate)

Henry's days and nights once revolved around urination. At work he found himself hurrying to the bathroom every hour. On airplanes or in theaters he picked aisle seats close to the restroom. Nights were the worst. "I was getting up five or six times a night to relieve myself," says the sixty-six-year-old retired chemical engineer. After months of procrastination and several lectures from his wife, he went to see a urologist. "I was afraid I had cancer. When he told me it was just a common problem called BPH I almost cried with relief."

Henry has benign prostatic hyperplasia, a gradual enlargement of the prostate that occurs in most men over the age of fifty. Had he mentioned prostate trouble at work or in a group of friends, odds are he would have met several fellow sufferers. An estimated 20 million men, most of them over the age of sixty, have an enlarging prostate, making it the most common medical problem plaguing older men.

Before going any further, two key points must be stressed about benign prostatic hyperplasia:

- *It is not cancer,* does not become cancer, and does not make a man more susceptible to developing prostate cancer. The same proportion of men *with* symptomatic BPH develop prostate cancer—about one in ten—as those *without* BPH.
- *It is not a life-threatening problem.* In the United States, fewer than two men of every 100,000 die from BPH, fewer than die from sports-related injuries. According to a panel of nationally recognized experts, "BPH affects the *quality* rather than the *quantity* of life."

What Is BPH?

Instead of shrinking with age, your prostate actually grows and becomes more muscular. This added tissue invariably presses into the urethra, reducing the diameter of the urine-carrying tube. Thus the symptoms of this condition are usually linked with urination. Unfortunately, many men chalk up their urinary changes to "getting older" and suffer needlessly, not taking advantage of treatments that could give them welcome relief. Or BPH can be mistaken for other common problems, including prostate cancer, diabetes, prostatitis, or urinary tract infection.

Virtually all the classic symptoms of BPH involve urination. Some men have just one symptom, others a whole constellation. Here is a list of the most common ones, labeled with the short-hand term that physicians generally use to describe them:

- *Impaired stream.* A noticeably slower or less forceful urine stream.

• *Hesitancy*. You have to stand at the urinal for a while before beginning to urinate. Some men find themselves waiting thirty seconds or more before their urine begins to flow.

• *Incomplete emptying*. The minute you've finished urinating, zip up your pants, and start washing your hands, your bladder feels full again and you have to go back and start over.

• *Terminal dribbling*. Instead of finishing with a strong flow and a squirt or two to empty your bladder, your urine slowly tapers off and drips uncontrollably from your penis. This dripping can last for a minute or longer.

• *Frequency*. You find yourself in the bathroom more often than you used to, and the intervals between each urination are shorter. Instead of once every two to three hours, you're urinating once every hour or less.

• *Nocturia*. Being awakened at night with the sudden and demanding urge to urinate. This may happen three, four, or more times a night.

• *Urgency*. When you need to go, you really need to go! Men with urgency say that the need to urinate appears suddenly and can't easily be delayed. Sometimes the urge comes on so quickly, and with such insistence, that you involuntarily urinate into your shorts before getting to the toilet. (This is called urge incontinence.)

While these are the classic symptoms, other ailments can also signal the presence of BPH. These include lower back pain, a little blood in the urine, or the sudden inability to urinate at all.

What Causes BPH

Exactly why the prostate begins to enlarge after years of no growth remains a mystery. So far, scientists have identified two conditions that are absolutely essential for BPH to develop—functioning testes that produce testosterone and some as-yet-undiscovered aging factor.

Men who have had their testes removed at an early age (because of cancer or another problem) never develop BPH, nor do men with congenital diseases that keep testosterone production low or switched off completely. The connection is so ironclad that removing the testes, an operation known as an orchiectomy or castration, was once used to treat severe BPH. Once the testosterone-making machinery has been removed, the prostate invariably shrinks to a near-normal size.

Age also plays a crucial role. Autopsies of several thousand men who died suddenly (in car accidents, of heart attacks, etc.) show that less than 5 percent of men under age forty have signs of prostatic hyperplasia. That number rises to 50 percent of men over age sixty, and 90 percent of those over age eighty-five. Bear in mind, though, that only a fraction of men with an enlarged prostate experience the symptoms of this condition.

Although the *why* of BPH remains murky, the *how* of it is coming to light. Some natural signal stimulates cells in the transition zone—that part of the prostate wrapped directly around the urethra—to grow and divide. At the same time, older cells linger longer than they normally should and don't die off when their time is up. The net effect of these actions transforms the transition zone from approximately 5 percent of the prostate's volume to as much as 50 percent in a man with severe BPH. The bulk of this growth occurs right around the flexible urethra.

This growth is called *benign* to set it apart from *malignant*, or cancerous, growth. New cells in the BPH growth region retain all the characteristics of normal prostate cells. They look like prostate cells. They manufacture the right hormones and secrete them into seminal fluid. They develop into tiny glands and muscle fibers. More important, new cells formed by BPH stay put in the prostate. Malignant cells, by comparison, eventually stop acting like prostate cells. They form disorganized tumors instead of organized glands. And they break away and wander to other parts of the body, a process called metastasis.

If the prostate gland were infinitely expandable, its middle-aged spread wouldn't cause urinary problems. But it isn't. So it does. As described in Chapter 1, a band of muscle and dense tissue surrounds the prostate. This capsule checks the gland's outward expansion and holds it in, much like the leather jacket on a football prevents the rubber bladder inside from getting too large. Since the new tissue must go somewhere, it pushes inward around the urethral space. The larger the transition zone grows, the smaller the urethra becomes. It can narrow from the diameter of a dime to that of a cocktail straw.

That's where the trouble starts. BPH or no BPH, you still generate the same amount of urine every hour—more if you spend a lazy afternoon fishing and drinking beer. Only now it must pass through a narrower tube on its way from bladder to penis. And that means a slower, less forceful stream.

The body doesn't necessarily accept these changes without a fight. To start urine flowing more quickly or to keep the stream moving along at more than a trickle, men often consciously or subconsciously contract the muscles that squeeze the bladder. This generates substantial pressure inside the bladder and puts more force behind the urine stream, often enough to pry open the urethra. (It's basically the same principle you apply when squeezing a beach ball or air mattress to deflate it faster.) This does the trick for the moment, but it ultimately makes the problem worse. Working the muscle around the bladder builds it up the same way that lifting weights builds biceps. Unfortunately, this extra muscle cuts down on the bladder's volume, so it holds less liquid. Less urine-storing capacity translates into more frequent trips to the bathroom. In addition, this new muscle responds to stimulation more readily than normal bladder muscle and sometimes contracts on its own. Such sudden and unexpected spasms can start urine flowing without any warning, giving rise to an urgent need to urinate.

Given the inevitability of BPH, are there any steps you can take to prevent it? So far scientists haven't discovered any risk factors that predispose a man to prostate enlargement. Sexual promiscuity, sexual abstinence, having a first ejaculation before age twelve, not having a first ejaculation until after age eighteen, smoking, diet, occupation—none appears to cause BPH.

Diagnosing BPH

Hesitancy, frequency, urgency, and awakening at night to urinate can all arise for a variety of reasons. In addition to an accurate medical history—your own description of symptoms and how you've been feeling—several tests will help pinpoint BPH and rule out other problems such as prostate cancer or diabetes.

• During a digital rectal exam, an enlarged prostate feels much like a normal prostate, though larger. A cancer-containing prostate, by comparison, may contain a hard lump or nodule. Acute bacterial prostatitis swells the prostate but makes it feel on the mushy side, and often painful to the touch.

• A blood test called the prostate-specific-antigen test (PSA) may also help. PSA is a protein made primarily by prostate cells—normal, hyperplastic, or malignant (cancerous) cells. In the healthy prostate, this protein is stored inside the gland and released into seminal fluid at ejaculation; only minute amounts ever enter the bloodstream. Anything below 4.0 nanograms of PSA per milliliter of blood is generally considered normal, though the cutoff for normal increases with age. But BPH, prostate infection, or a tumor either signals prostate cells to make more of this protein, or makes the gland "leaky," causing PSA to end up in the bloodstream.

Tumor cells manufacture far more PSA than do BPH cells. Researchers estimate that one gram of BPH tissue increases PSA values by about 0.3 (0.30 nanograms PSA per milliliter of blood) while one gram of tumor increases PSA levels by 3.5. Physicians have begun applying this difference by calculating what they call PSA density: the ratio of PSA to prostate volume. The smaller this number, the more likely the elevated PSA is due to BPH, while high PSA densities suggest prostate cancer. Prostate size can be measured with relative accuracy using transrectal ultrasound (see Chapter 6).

• Another blood test, this one for a protein called serum creatinine, can spot kidney problems that often occur as part of the BPH "chain reaction." A nearly-always-filled bladder can generate enough back pressure to slow the flow of urine through the ureters, the tubes connecting each kidney with the bladder. If the blockage is severe enough or extends over a long period of time, one or both kidneys may begin failing. Creatinine is a waste product normally excreted in urine, so above-normal levels in the blood can indicate kidney distress.

• A urine test can rule out infection as a cause of urinary symptoms. This involves nothing more than washing your hands, cleaning the head of your penis with an antiseptic wipe, and urinating into a sterile plastic cup. Bacteria or sediment in the urine suggest an infection that can usually be treated with antibiotics (see Chapter 2). While the absence of bacteria doesn't prove that urinary symptoms are caused by BPH, it does point in that direction.

• A series of seven questions (fig. 3.1) developed by the American Urological Association (AUA) helps determine how much the symptoms of BPH disturb your life. The lower the score, the lower the "bothersomeness." In fact, most urologists use this scale to assess a man's symptoms and determine appropriate treatment. A 0 to 7 score indicates mild prostate disease, 8 to 18 indicates moderate disease, and 19 to 35 means severe BPH. Figure 3.2 suggests possible treatment options for each stage.

A panel of experts assembled by the federal Agency for Health Care Policy Research recently published guidelines to help physicians diagnose and treat BPH. Their report, coauthored by Dr. Michael Barry, a Massachusetts General Hospital (MGH) internist and coleader of a national prostate disease study team, says the five tests described above are almost always sufficient to accurately identify BPH. For men with the most severe symptoms, or those with nerve damage or suspected bladder cancer or other problems, additional tests might be necessary. These include:

Figure 3.1. AUA Symptom Index

Questions to be answered	Not at all	Less than 1 time in 5	Less than half the time	About half the time	More than half the time	Almost always
			AUA Symptom Score (Circle 1 number on each line)			
1. Over the past month, how often have you had a sensation of not emptying your bladder completely after you finished urinating?	0	1	2	3	4	5
2. Over the past month, how often have you had to urinate again less than 2 hours after you finished urinating?	0	1	2	3	4	5
3. Over the past month, how often have you found you stopped and started again several times when you urinated?	0	1	2	3	4	5
4. Over the past month, how often have you found it difficult to postpone urination?	0	1	2	3	4	5
5. Over the past month, how often have you had a weak urinary stream?	0	1	2	3	4	5
6. Over the past month, how often have you had to push or strain to begin urination?	0	1	2	3	4	5
7. Over the past month, how many times did you most typically get up to urinate from the time you went to bed at night until the time you got up in the morning?	0 (None)	1 (1 time)	2 (2 times)	3 (3 times)	4 (4 times)	5 (5 times or more)

Sum of 7 circled numbers (AUA Symptom Score): _____

SOURCE: Barry, Fowler, O'Leary et al. "The American Urological Association Symptom Index for Benign Prostatic Hyperplasic." *Journal of Urology* 1992, 148:1549–57. Used with permission.

- Uroflowmetry, urinating as normally as possible (in the privacy of a medical office bathroom, of course!) into a special toilet that measures the amount of urine voided each second as well as average and peak rates of urination. These numbers sometimes help physicians tell the difference between BPH and a nerve problem that may be interfering with urination.

- Cystoscopy, a procedure in which a physician inserts a flexible tube with a tiny camera and light into the urethra. This allows him or her to inspect the urethra, which forms the inner border of the prostate, and the bladder. Small tumors, narrowings of the urethra, and other anomalies that might interfere with urination can be detected this way.

Figure 3.2. Treatment options for BPH depending upon the severity of symptoms

TREATMENT	SEVERITY OF PROSTATISM (SYMPTOM SCORE*)			
	MILD (0–7)	MODERATE (8–18)	SEVERE (19–35)	WITH URINARY RETENTION
Watchful waiting	Yes	Yes	No	No
5α-Reductase inhibitors	No	Yes	Yes	No
α1-Adrenergic antagonists	No	Yes	Yes	No
Microwave therapy	No	Yes	Yes	No
Laser prostatectomy	No	Yes	Yes	No
Prostatic stents	No	Yes	Yes	Yes
Transurethral incision of the prostate	No	Yes	Yes	Yes
Transurethral resection of the prostate	No	Yes	Yes	Yes
Open prostatectomy	No	No	Yes	Yes

SOURCE: JE Oesterling, "Benign Prostatic Hyperplasia." *New England Journal of Medicine* 1995, 332:99–109. Used with permission.

*Symptom scores are as determined with the American Urological Association questionnaire shown in Figure 3.1.

Computerized tomography (CT) scans and magnetic resonance imaging (MRI) scans, both accurate but expensive ways to see into the body, give a physician very little useful information when it comes to an uncomplicated case of BPH, the panel concluded. So if your physician schedules one of these, you might want to ask why.

Treating BPH

While the vast majority of men over fifty have enlarging prostates, fewer than half of them become aware of this natural phenomenon. And only 5 percent or so become irritated enough by their symptoms to seek out treatment. Currently there's no way to predict which men will be bothered by BPH. There's little connection between how large a man's prostate becomes and the onset or severity of urinary symptoms. Some men whose prostates double in size remain blissfully unaware of that growth. Others develop moderate to severe symptoms with only a small increase in prostate size.

Thankfully, several strategies have been developed for treating the symptoms of BPH: watchful waiting, drug therapy, surgery, balloon dilation, and a few still-experimental techniques. Should you immediately seek treatment at the first sign of BPH? Probably not. Though effective, most treatments have side effects that could overwhelm the benefits of the relief they offer.

One of the first early signs that men notice connected to benign prostate growth is having to get up at night to urinate. Men often come into my office very alarmed they're getting up once or twice a night to go to the bathroom. I tell them that the average sixty-year-old man gets up at least once a night. Just hearing that this is normal often gives a man a tremendous amount of relief. Many don't really need treatment and are quite content to live with these minor symptoms.

The key question that can help you decide on treatment is this: Do the symptoms caused by an enlarged prostate bother you? If they don't, then why have surgery or take drugs every day? If, however, urinary symptoms caused by BPH make you miserable or interfere with work, pleasure, and sleep, then by all means take the plunge. This is where the AUA Symptom Index comes in. If you aren't particularly bothered by your symptoms, or score 7 or less on the AUA scale, you might try watchful waiting, sometimes called expectant monitoring. It costs no more than the price of a visit to your physician every six to twelve months. More important, it carries zero risk for treatment-related complications, which can include incontinence, dizziness, and ejaculatory problems. And if your symptoms get worse, then it's easy to move on to more aggressive treatment. If, on the other hand, urinary symptoms fragment your sleep or you find yourself standing in front of a urinal far too often during the day, drug therapy or surgery may offer welcome relief. Unfortunately, neither option *guarantees* relief.

Ask your physician for an opinion on which treatments are medically appropriate for you. If you have a serious heart condition, for example, he or she might not recommend surgery. If you've had an episode of urinary retention—the inability to urinate, usually treated by inserting a catheter through the urethra or abdomen into the bladder to drain out the accumulated urine—surgery may offer the most permanent relief.

"If several options look feasible, then your own preferences should play a major role in making the decision," says Dr. Barry. Perhaps you don't relish the thought of taking a pill a day for years, or you don't want to risk even the remote possibility of incontinence. Don't be afraid to speak up and tell your physician what your goals and priorities are.

Watchful Waiting

Despite the official title, watchful waiting is really a slightly advanced version of what men have been doing for years—living with their symptoms and hoping they'll either go away or, at the very least, not get much worse. Throw in regular, objective evaluations by a physician and procrastination becomes a medically sound approach recently backed by the blue-ribbon panel of BPH experts assembled by the Agency for Health Care Policy Research.

Watchful waiting offers men with tolerable BPH symptoms several advantages. It requires nothing more of a man than monitoring his symptoms and seeing his physician once or twice a year—no drug-taking, no hospital stay, no recovery from surgery and days lost from work. Watchful waiting doesn't increase a man's risk of dying from treatment-related complications or suffering because of them. Nor does it increase his chances of becoming incontinent, impotent, or infertile, as do more aggressive treatments. Since the symptoms of BPH don't inevitably progress, up to 50 percent of all men who try watchful waiting never get worse, and some—about 5 to 10 percent—even see their urinary symptoms spontaneously diminish.

The point of watchful waiting is not to see how long you can go without treatment. In fact, delaying too long after symptoms have worsened can lead to potentially irreversible kidney damage. The key is checking with your physician when you notice a suspicious change. Meanwhile, several simple changes in your daily routine can potentially reduce the irritating symptoms:

• To reduce the number of times you have to urinate at night, try not drinking any fluids between dinner and bedtime.
• During the day, avoid beverages like coffee, tea, beer, wine, and liquor. All contain diuretics, compounds that increase urine production.
• If a sudden urge to urinate seems to strike every two hours, go to the bathroom every one and one-half hours, so you aren't caught up short.
• Avoid antihistamines and over-the-counter cold remedies that contain pseudoephedrine, such as Sudafed, Nyquil, and others. They tend to contract the pelvic floor muscles and urethra, further narrowing the space for urination.

The only real drawback of watchful waiting is the small chance that prostate enlargement will suddenly block urine flow through the urethra. Such complete obstruction can be quite frightening and a bit painful. But it is easily fixed in your physician's office or a hospital emergency room. A catheter inserted into the bladder can quickly release the pent-up urine. Aggressive therapy such as a transurethral resection of the prostate (see page 44) usually follows an event like this.

Drug Therapy

You can take drugs to quiet angina, lower cholesterol, or control blood pressure. What about a pill for the prostate? Since ancient times, healers and charlatans have prescribed a cornucopia of plant potions for "starting the urine" and relieving BPH. These include stinging nettle, pumpkin seeds, aspen, and rye, to name a few. An extract made from berries of the saw palmetto tree, which grows in the southeastern United States, is sold as a natural remedy for BPH. Several clinical trials in Europe indicate that this extract, marketed under the name Pro-Sanoa, may indeed relieve symptoms. But since the symptoms of BPH can improve on their own, some researchers suggest this extract may be little more than an expensive way of delivering a placebo.

Two officially sanctioned medical treatments appeared in the United States at the beginning of this decade. Each hits a completely different BPH target; each has a unique activity profile and range of side effects. So a man who cannot take one may be able to take the other, or one of several even newer drugs that should be on the market soon.

Drug therapy is certainly less invasive than surgery, balloon dilation, or hyperthermia. It requires no hospital stay, no catheterization, no chance of treatment-related infection or incontinence. So why isn't it the number-one choice for treating BPH? Physicians are rightfully cautious when faced with a new treatment. While drug therapy appears to relieve the symptoms of BPH in some men, it hasn't been used long enough to determine what, if any, the long-term effects may be. Demand from men, however, is increasing the popularity of this approach. While roughly 20 percent of men initially tried drug therapy for BPH symptoms in 1993, as many as 50 percent are expected to try it by the late 1990s.

Drug therapy doesn't work for all men. This probably stems from the fact that urinary symptoms resulting from BPH appear for different reasons—increased pressure on the urethra, weakening of the bladder neck, bladder-muscle hyperstimulation, or something else. Not all of these may respond to the same drugs.

Alpha-Blockers

New prostate tissue formed by benign hyperplasia is rich in smooth muscle. This resembles the muscles lining blood vessels and intestines more than it resembles triceps or thighs. Smooth muscle is controlled by the autonomic nervous system, which also controls heartbeat, breathing, blood pressure, and a host of automatic activities. It contracts when signaled by tiny chemical transmitters circulating in the bloodstream. Drugs called alpha-blockers relax smooth muscle by preventing these transmitters from attaching to receptors on the cells' surface.

Alpha-blockers have been used for years to treat men and women with high blood pressure. The drugs relax the smooth muscle that lines arteries, opening them up to permit greater blood flow. The first alpha-blocker approved for treating BPH, called terazosin, began its medical life as a drug for high blood pressure. Terazosin (Hytrin) appears to work on two fronts. It relaxes the smooth muscle in the prostate itself, opening the urethral channel. It also relaxes smooth muscle in the bladder, making it contract and spasm less often. This can quell the urgent need to urinate that accompanies BPH.

Alpha-blockers diminish urinary symptoms in more than half the men who try them. (While terazosin is the most common, several others are also being investigated or used. These include doxazosin (Cardura), tamsulosin, and alfuzosin.) It usually takes two to three weeks to notice a change, and rarely takes longer than twelve weeks.

Finding the right dose can be tricky. Since the drug circulates to every tissue, it alters smooth muscle function throughout the body. Taking too large a dose can cause dizziness or even fainting when a man stands up, a condition known as postural hypotension. Too much alpha-blocker can also cause headaches, fatigue, and nasal congestion. Most men are started on the lowest daily dose possible and gradually work their way up to find the optimal dose—one that reduces symptoms the most and generates the fewest side effects. All of the side effects subside once the drug is discontinued. However, men for whom an alpha-blocker keeps BPH symptoms under control will likely use the drug for life. Terazosin won FDA approval for treating BPH in 1993, so few men have taken it for very long. However, people have taken similar alpha-blockers for years for other conditions with few long-term side effects.

5-alpha-reductase Inhibitors

For years testosterone has been fingered as the bad guy in the BPH story. Men who produce no testosterone, such as those born without functioning testes or those castrated later in life, are never troubled by an enlarged prostate. But testosterone itself may not be the culprit. Inside the prostate, an enzyme modifies this hormone just a little, forming a new compound called 5-dihydrotestosterone. DHT, for short, appears to be the real trigger for stimulating hyperplastic growth in the prostate. If a drug could block this conversion, scientists reasoned, it might prevent BPH or possibly shrink the prostate enough to relieve symptoms.

In 1984, researchers discovered the compound finasteride. In test tubes it prevented the enzyme 5-alpha reductase from turning testosterone into 5-DHT. Experiments with old beagles suffering from BPH, and then clinical trials with several hundred men, showed that finasteride could decrease 5-DHT levels inside the prostate.

Extensive testing in the United States and abroad involved more than 1,500 volunteers with BPH. In half the men, daily doses of finasteride (Proscar) shrank prostate size an average of 20 percent and significantly improved urinary symptoms. In the other half it had little or no effect. The only important side effect was temporary impotence, loss of sex drive, or abnormal ejaculations in about 5 percent of the volunteers, compared to 1.5 percent of those taking a placebo. Both potency and libido returned soon after the men stopped taking the drug.

The main drawback of finasteride treatment is that it takes up to six months to see any improvement. That's fine for the men in whom it does work. But it is frustrating for others who take the drug for six months only to find out it has no effect for them. As physicians follow patients taking finasteride or other 5-alpha-reductase inhibitors soon to arrive on the market, they hope to find ways to identify which men will benefit from this drug therapy and which men won't.

One other potential drawback is that these drugs reduce PSA levels, and may make detection of prostate cancer a bit tricky. As a general rule, a 5-alpha-reductase inhibitor like finasteride will drop a man's PSA level 50 percent, though in reality that reduction ranges from 30 percent to 80 percent. To be on the safe side, it's probably wise to have a PSA test once you've been taking finasteride or another 5-alpha-reductase inhibitor for several months to establish a new baseline value. From then on, anything above that level could suggest the possibility of tumor growth.

Surgery

Surgery offers the most reliable method for improving BPH-related symptoms. Four procedures—transurethral resection of the prostate, transurethral incision of the prostate, transurethral laser incision of the prostate, and open prostatectomy—are safe, effective, and widely used. The transurethral resection, or TURP, is by far the most popular, with about 400,000 performed each year. That makes it the second most common operation after cataract surgery in men over sixty-five. But common or popular does not necessarily mean best. In the recent national guidelines about BPH, the experts suggest that transurethral incision of the prostate is just as effective for certain men, has fewer complications, and has shorter hospitalization and recovery times. They call it an underused procedure that should be more widely practiced.

All surgical procedures can lead to unwanted and unavoidable complications. These are no different (fig. 3.3). Before agreeing to an operation, make sure you discuss the advantages and disadvantages with your surgeon and your physician. Ask about the potential for complications in general and whether you have any medical conditions that might increase the odds.

While any surgeon can perform these procedures, it's best to get your care from a board-certified urologist. These physicians have satisfied demanding requirements set by the American Board of Urology and qualify as specialists in treating diseases of the male urinary and reproductive system. The success of any operation depends in

Figure 3.3. BPH treatment outcomes

Treatment Outcomes	Surgical Options			Non-Surgical Options		
	TUIP	TURP	Open Surgery	Watchful Waiting	Alpha Blocker	Finasteride
Chance for improvement of symptoms	80%	90%	95%	10%	70%	60%
Degree of symptom improvement (% reduction in symptom score)	70%	80%	85%		50%	30%
Morbidity/complications (20% of these are significant—the remainder are minor)	10%	15%	20%	3%	15%	15%
Chance of dying within 90 days of treatment	1%	1.5%	2%	0.8% chance of death within 90 days for a 67-year-old man		
Risk of total urinary incontinence	0.1%	0.5%	0.5%	Minimal chance with all forms of treatment		
Need for operative treatment to correct surgical complications	1%	4%	4%	N/A	N/A	N/A
Risk of impotence	5%	10%	10%	2–5% for all forms of medical therapy		
Risk of retrograde ejaculation	30%	95%	95%	0	10%	0
Loss of work time (days)	7	7	14–21	1	4	2
Hospital stay	0–1	1–3	5–7			

SOURCE: JE Oesterling, "Benign Prostatic Hyperplasia." *New England Journal of Medicine* 1995, 332:99–109. Used with permission.

large part on a surgeon's skill, and skill is often a function of experience. Ask your physician how many of these operations he or she has done before, or how many he or she does a month. Also ask about his or her complication rate. Don't let anyone hurry you into the operation. Since BPH isn't a life-threatening condition, you have plenty of time. Ask some questions, read up on the subject, and then ask more questions. If a potential surgeon is reluctant to talk with you or tries to rush you through this stage of your investigation, that may be an indicator of how he or she will treat you after the surgery. Though skill is critical, compassion and understanding count for a great deal as well. Take the time to get a second opinion if you feel you need one.

Transurethral Resection of the Prostate (TURP)

Men who have had this operation regularly refer to it as the "reaming out" or "Roto-Rooter" procedure. Though unscientific, the terms vividly and accurately describe the intent of a transurethral resection of the prostate, or TURP for short: removing ingrown prostate tissue from around the urethral space, opening this channel to allow urine to flow through it more freely. The operation's popularity stems from its effectiveness—it relieves urinary symptoms in approximately 70 percent of the men who undergo it. Its simplicity, relatively low complication rate, and relatively short recovery period also add to its appeal.

TURPs are closed procedures, meaning the surgeon makes no incision to get at the prostate. Instead, he or she removes excess prostate tissue through the penis using a device called a resectoscope. This versatile, crayon-thick tool carries a lens system, a bright light, an irrigation tube

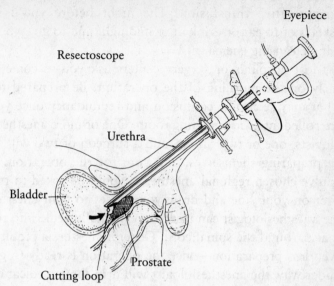

Figure 3.4. *A surgeon slides the resectoscope through the urethra and into the prostate. Looking through the eyepiece, he or she can position the cutting loop and remove parts of the gland that may be obstructing the urethra.*

and a cutting tool (fig. 3.4). It is inserted into the penis and then slid through the urethra until it is positioned inside the prostate. Performing a TURP is like removing the pulp from an orange without disturbing the peel. First, tissue is removed to open the central tube. Then that opening is enlarged, making an unobstructed conduit for urine without ever disturbing the prostate's outer coat.

Preparing for a TURP takes relatively little time. A few weeks in advance you'll go in for some baseline tests, such as an electrocardiogram to check your heart, a battery of blood tests, and a talk with an anesthesiologist. You may wish to bank one or two units of blood several weeks before the operation, since about one in ten men require a postoperative transfusion. The night before you'll be asked not to eat or drink after midnight and to give yourself a cleansing enema.

Most hospitals or surgery centers ask you to come in early on the morning of the operation. Be prepared for what may seem like confusion and redundancy once you are rolled into the operating room. One or more anesthesiologists, one or two nurses, and a surgeon or two will all be preparing themselves, and you, for the operation. If you've chosen regional anesthesia, you'll be asked to roll over on your side and draw your knees to your chest so the anesthesiologist can insert a very small needle into the space around the spinal cord. General anesthesia requires even less preparation—once the operation is ready to get under way, the anesthesiologist will drip some medication into the intravenous tube in your arm and you will instantly fall asleep.

Once the anesthesia kicks in, the surgeon generously lubricates the inside of the penis and the outside of the resectoscope. He or she then inserts the device into the tip of the urethra and gently works it into the prostate. Looking through the lens, he or she inspects the walls of the urethra, the overgrown prostate tissue, blood vessels, muscles, and other important landmarks. Once everything is in place, the surgeon presses a trigger on the resectoscope, which moves a wire loop back and forth. Another button sends a current of electricity through the loop, heating it up. Using this heat scalpel, the surgeon shaves small strips of prostate away from the urethral space. Little pressure is needed—the loop slides through the tissue like a hot knife through butter.

The loop also performs another important task. On a different power setting it cauterizes, or seals off, blood vessels ruptured when prostate tissue is removed. Bleeding is easily controlled during this procedure, so the majority of men don't require a transfusion during or after the hour-long procedure.

Once a smooth channel for urine has been created and all bleeding stopped, the surgeon flushes out the bladder with sterile cleansing fluid. This washes out all the prostate shavings or chips. They are collected, preserved, and later examined under a microscope for signs of early prostate cancer. A TURP turns up signs of prostate cancer in about one in ten men.

To complete the TURP, the surgeon places a Foley catheter into the bladder. This is essentially a long, sterile rubber tube with a small, deflated balloon on one end and a bag on the other (fig. 3.5). The balloon end is slid into the penis, through the urethra and into the bladder. Once in place, the balloon is inflated and sealed shut. This creates a collar much too large to fit through the bladder neck or the urethra, anchoring the catheter in place. The other end hangs from the penis and attaches to a bag for catching and collecting urine (see fig. 3.6.).

The Foley catheter has several functions. For the first few hours after surgery, sterile water is flushed into the catheter. This dilutes any blood leaking from unsealed vessels and prevents blood clots. More important, the catheter drains urine directly out of the bladder, bypassing the newly formed channel and protecting it from irritating chemicals in urine.

The average post-TURP hospital stay lasts two days. You'll probably be eating food the evening of your operation and will almost certainly walk around your room or up and down the hospital corridors. Walking with a Foley catheter in place takes some getting used to, but can easily

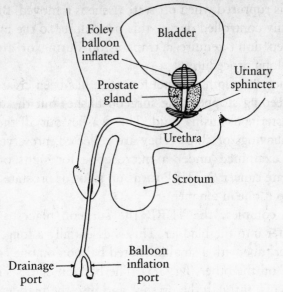

Foley balloon inflated

Bladder

Prostate gland

Urinary sphincter

Urethra

Scrotum

Drainage port

Balloon inflation port

Figure 3.5. *A Foley catheter is used to drain urine out of the bladder. The catheter is inserted into the tip of the urethra and gently slid into the bladder. Once in place, a small balloon is inflated, preventing the catheter from sliding out.*

be mastered. The collection bag can be hung on a metal pole with wheels used for hanging intravenous fluid bags. The Foley will feel as if it is going to fall out at any moment. Don't worry—it won't. Once the fluid draining from your penis and bladder is clear of blood, the Foley will be removed. Opening a valve allows the fluid-filled ball anchoring it inside the bladder to deflate, and the whole tube slides out of the penis.

TURPs often provide almost immediate relief of urinary symptoms, though some men must wait a month or two to reap the benefits. About 95 percent of men who undergo a TURP report a noticeable decrease in their BPH-related symptoms. The effects last a lifetime for some men.

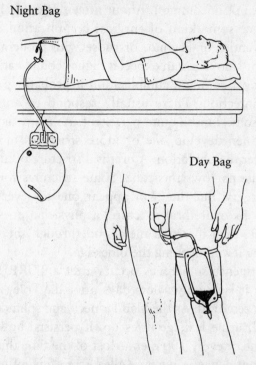

Figure 3.6. *You can connect different kinds of collection bags to a Foley catheter. The larger night bag can be hung from a bed or chair. A smaller day bag can be strapped to your leg. It's invisible underneath pants.*

But occasionally a repeat TURP is needed, sometimes in as little as three to five years.

The TURP isn't a cost-free miracle procedure, and the potential complications merit some serious thought. About one in every 100 men who have a TURP die within ninety days of the surgery. These are usually older men, or smokers, or men with bad hearts, failing livers, or other health problems. Still, some otherwise healthy men do die as a result of their TURPs. Less drastic surgical complications are not uncommon. About fifteen of every 100 men experience some kind of surgical complication. Men in their seventies or beyond, or those with moderate heart disease or smokers, can expect a higher complication rate.

The most common complication is probably a postoperative infection. These usually respond to antibiotics, though some can be quite persistent. As many as 10 percent of men develop one or more strictures months or years after the operation. A urethral stricture occurs when scar tissue narrows this tube. Some strictures form soon after surgery, but they can appear one to several years later. To fix a urethral stricture, a physician anesthetizes the penis, then inserts a metal rod through the urethra, stretching it and opening the blockage.

Incontinence sometimes occurs after a TURP. Most of the time it lasts only a few days after the Foley catheter has been removed. As the bladder neck and sphincter muscles heal, urine leakage dries up. It persists, however, in about one of every 100 men. Most of the time this persistent incontinence is what's called stress incontinence—a small squirt of urine expelled when a man sneezes, laughs, sits down, or does some other activity that compresses the bladder. Exercises that strengthen the sphincter can help overcome this annoying and potentially embarrassing problem (see Chapter 13). If the bladder neck or sphincter muscle is inadvertently damaged during the operation, a more constant incontinence is possible.

A TURP can also interfere with sexual function. Up to 30 percent of men report impotence following the procedure. This figure may be an overestimate, because no one really knows what proportion of men are impotent *before* surgery. No studies have ever determined how many men become impotent because of a TURP, and how many blame aging-associated impotence on their surgery. Men who are potent going into a TURP usually regain their potency once they've healed. A transurethral resection can cause impotence by damaging the nerves that control the blood vessels and penile tissues involved in creating an erection. It does not, however, reduce a man's desire for sex—his libido—or his capacity for sexual pleasure. A man with TURP-related impotence can still have an orgasm. (Chapter 13 describes a number of techniques available for impotent men who wish to maintain an active sex life.)

What many men *can't* do after a TURP, however, is ejaculate. To open a clear channel through the urethra, surgeons usually remove the zone of prostate tissue surrounding the upper end of the urethra, directly below the bladder. During orgasm, this muscular tissue contracts around the very top of the urethra, clamping it closed and directing sperm and seminal fluid down and out the penis. Removing this tissue keeps the bladder neck open, allowing seminal fluid to flow into the bladder. Nothing comes out of the penis at orgasm. These backward, or retrograde, ejaculations feel much the same as normal ones, but they are dry.

A man who needs a TURP but also hopes to someday father a child has three options he can pursue. He can hope that the procedure does not cause retrograde ejaculations. He can store his sperm before the operation at a medical center or private cryogenic facility. These are often listed in the Yellow Pages under "sperm bank." Semen frozen in liquid nitrogen to a chilly –196 degrees Celsius can be thawed out months or years later and used in one of several artificial insemination techniques. The third option involves flushing out the bladder with a catheter immediately after ejaculation, collecting the liquid and separating out the sperm to be used later during artificial insemination. This is usually done at a center specializing in reproductive problems.

Physicians generally assume that by the time a man develops BPH, his child-raising days are over. Few ever raise the subject of infertility. If your physician doesn't bring up the subject of sexuality or fertility, and you have questions, *ask*. You have the right to know all the consequences of a procedure.

Second-Generation TURP Techniques

Several newer technologies have been developed to remove prostate tissue via the transurethral route. A new type of wire loop vaporizes BPH tissue rather than merely slicing through it. This causes far less bleeding and reduces the time a man spends in the hospital recuperating. The disadvantage is that no "chips" are removed that can be inspected for the signs of prostate cancer.

Another exciting advancement involves treating BPH with laser energy in a procedure called visual laser ablation of the prostate, or VLAP. Lasers are instruments that emit a precise beam of light energetic enough to destroy tissue. Some high-powered lasers are already used in surgery in place of scalpels; low-powered lasers are widely used to remove birthmarks and tattoos. For treating an enlarged prostate, a tiny laser is inserted into the urethra and aimed at the surrounding hyperplastic tissue. The laser light quickly kills prostate tissue. In most cases, the dead and dying tissue swells up before it breaks apart and is eliminated during urination. As a precaution, a small catheter is usually inserted through the lower abdomen directly into the bladder until any swelling subsides and normal urinary function returns.

Transurethral Incision of the Prostate (TUIP)

A less common procedure called transurethral incision of the prostate, or TUIP, can be as effective as transurethral resection of the prostate but is associated with fewer complications. It, too, is a closed procedure, performed with an instrument inserted into the penis and prostate. But instead of scraping away and removing pieces of prostate tissue, the surgeon uses a tiny blade at the tip of the instrument to make one or two cuts that run the length and depth of the gland. This opens up the prostate, relieving pressure on the urethra and improving urinary flow. Preparation for a TUIP is identical to that for a transurethral resection, as is postoperative care.

TUIP appears to be almost as effective as TURP in relieving urinary symptoms caused by an enlarging prostate. What's more, it leads to fewer surgical complications like incontinence and retrograde ejaculation (fig. 3.3). But not everyone is a candidate for TUIP or its experimental cousin, TULIP—transurethral laser incision of the prostate. Men with very large prostate glands or those with severe symptoms generally don't get much relief from these procedures and are better served by a TURP.

Several critics cite another drawback of TUIP and TULIP. Since no tissue is removed during the procedure, there's no chance to find microscopic evidence of early prostate cancer. That may be a minor drawback, since many of the tumors discovered this way are so small they don't require treatment. The no-tissue issue probably shouldn't deter you from choosing the procedure you want. Once it's over, you can still have an annual rectal exam and PSA test, an effective combination for detecting prostate cancer (see Chapter 6).

Open Simple Prostatectomy

For men with significant or clearly bothersome symptoms, or those with very large prostates, removing enlarged prostate tissue that's blocking the urethra by making a surgical incision may be the best course of action. This is a much more involved procedure than TURP or TUIP. It requires a three- to five-day hospital stay and several weeks of recovery. In addition, it is associated with higher rates of incontinence and impotence.

A simple prostatectomy removes only the benign growth that's throttling the urethra and leaves behind the gland itself, or at least the capsule and some tissue. The radical prostatectomy used to treat prostate cancer, in comparison, removes the entire prostate, a small section of the urethra, and the seminal vesicles.

Surgeons have developed two different techniques for a simple open prostatectomy. The suprapubic route approaches the prostate through an incision in the bladder, while the retropubic route approaches the benign tissue through an incision in the prostate itself. The one that's right for you depends on the size and shape of your prostate, other anatomic features, and your surgeon's own preference and experience.

A simple open prostatectomy removes the same zone of tissue as is removed during a TURP. Then why not always do the TURP, which requires no incisions and a shorter hospital stay? It takes too long to perform a TURP on a man with a very large prostate, increasing the risk of complications. In such cases the open procedure minimizes these risks and also increases the likelihood the urologist will remove virtually all of the offending BPH tissue.

As with a TURP, any remaining BPH tissue can continue growing. In some men this causes another round of urinary symptoms and perhaps another operation. It appears, though, that men who have a simple open prostatectomy don't require another operation as often as those who choose a TURP.

Since the prostate capsule remains intact, the likelihood of impotence or incontinence is not nearly as high with a simple open prostatectomy as it is with a radical prostatectomy. In fact, incontinence and impotence rates appear to be roughly the same for a TURP as they are for a simple prostatectomy.

Balloon Dilation

Rather than remove excess tissue or cut a slit in the prostate, some urologists use a small, powerful balloon to open up a BPH-narrowed urethra. The technique isn't new. French and British physicians in the mid-1800s fashioned metal rods for forcing open the urethral channel. In the 1830s, balloons used for making gold jewelry were attached to hollow tubes, inserted in the urethra, and then inflated, stretching the urethra and making urination easier. The equipment used today is more carefully and anatomically designed, but the principle is the same. Air pressure compresses and rearranges prostate tissue, pushing it away from the urethra and opening a larger unobstructed channel for urine.

The procedure is simpler, faster, and leads to complica-

tions in a smaller percentage of men than does transurethral resection of the prostate. In most hospitals it is
performed as a day surgery. A man arrives early in the
morning, goes to the operating room (after filling out all
the necessary paperwork, of course!), has the procedure,
and ends the day at home in his own bed.

Since no cutting or scraping is involved, balloon dilation is usually done under local anesthesia. Once the penis
has been anesthetized and lubricated, a flexible tube bearing a balloon on one end is inserted into the penis and
gently threaded into the prostate. The surgeon positions
the balloon by feeling it through the rectum, looking at it
through a lens system called a cystoscope, or taking an X
ray. Once the device is in place, the balloon is inflated to a
predetermined size, usually the width of your thumb.
After ten minutes or so, the surgeon deflates the balloon,
removes the dilator, and inserts a Foley catheter through
the urethra and into the bladder. This irrigates the bladder
and urethra, diluting any blood that might emerge from
broken blood vessels before it can clot. It also drains urine
directly out of the bladder, giving the newly opened and
potentially raw urethra two or three days to heal. Most
men go home with the catheter in place the day of their
surgery, and return to the urologist's office a few days
later to have it removed.

Compared to a TURP, balloon dilation has several advantages and drawbacks. It can be performed more
quickly and with fewer complications than a resection (fig.
3.3). The procedure generally leaves intact the zone of
highly contractile prostate tissue just below the bladder,
thus dramatically reducing the possibility of retrograde
ejaculation to under 5 percent. Balloon dilation rarely dis-
turbs the bladder sphincter muscle, so the rate of incontinence is below 1 percent.

However, it does not reduce urinary symptoms quite as effectively as TURP, open prostatectomy, TUIP, or TULIP. Only half of the men who choose the balloon procedure report a stronger, less hesitant urine stream or fewer trips to bathroom during the day and night, compared to 80 percent or more who choose surgery. It also appears that the symptoms of BPH return more quickly in some men who try balloon dilation. This isn't surprising, since the BPH tissue remains in place around the urethra. (A similar regrowth occurs after balloon angioplasty, a procedure used to open cholesterol-clogged arteries.) Too few men have been followed long enough after balloon dilation to make accurate statements about its long-term effect. It may be that regrowth occurs in a particular subgroup of men, such as those who have the worst pretreatment symptoms. Researchers are working to clear up this point, but it will take several years.

As urologists familiarize themselves with balloon dilation and examine their results, they're finding that the procedure isn't really meant for everyone with BPH. The best candidates appear to be men with smaller prostates, those whose symptoms aren't severe, and those who have not had an episode of urine retention. Good candidates may experience fewer side effects, report better improvement in symptoms, and require reoperation less frequently than described above.

Hyperthermia

Normal human cells withstand heat far better than tumor cells or hyperplastic cells such as those that cause BPH. Exploiting this difference, researchers have developed several ways of selectively killing abnormal cells while sparing normal tissue. The most widely tested of these, hyperthermia, uses microwaves to heat prostate tissue above 40 degrees Celsius.

Investigators have developed two separate routes for hyperthermia. In transurethral hyperthermia, the heating probe is housed in a thin tube that is slid into the penis and from there into the section of the urethra surrounded by the prostate. In transrectal hyperthermia, the probe is inserted into the rectum and positioned atop the nearby prostate. No matter what the route, the probe houses a small device that generates the same kind of microwaves as your kitchen microwave oven. Its purpose and method of operation are also identical. The probe generates very-high-frequency sound waves, far above the threshold of human hearing. These waves bounce into water-bearing tissue, excite the water molecules, and make them vibrate very quickly. As they slow down, the energy they give off appears as heat, which accumulates in the tissue.

The probe itself sits within a jacket of circulating cool water, which protects the urethra or rectum by keeping it at or near body temperature. The microwaves penetrate only a few centimeters into the prostate, exactly where the offending hyperplastic tissue resides. As the BPH cells heat up beyond their survival limit, they die off. The dead cells are either flushed out during urination or destroyed by the body's scavengers, white blood cells called macrophages.

Different treatment strategies have been investigated. One requires several sessions in which prostate tissue is heated to approximately 110 degrees F (44 degrees C). Another heats the prostate to between 130 degrees and 140 degrees F in a single session. So far, too few men have undergone microwave hyperthermia to realistically compare it with more standard, well-studied procedures. It appears to reduce symptoms somewhat less than TURP or

TUIP, and about the same as drug therapy. Complication and retreatment rates also appear to be low, but too few men have been followed for too short a period of time to accurately make this claim.

Stents

Miners learned centuries ago that the only way to keep an underground tunnel from collapsing was to prop it open with wood or rock columns. A similar concept has recently been extended to the urethral "tunnel." Researchers have implanted tiny tubes or coils called stents to prop open urethras that would otherwise be compressed by a growing prostate. While stents have not yet received FDA approval, several different types are being widely tested in the United States and Europe.

No surgery is needed to implant a stent. Regional anesthesia and intravenous painkillers are all that are needed to make the insertion pain-free. All an experienced urologist needs to do is slide a coiled-up or compressed stent into the urethra, guide it to the correct spot, and release it from its holder. The stent springs into place with enough force to open a permanent channel in the ever-narrowing urethra. The whole procedure takes about thirty minutes or less.

Stents offer several attractive advantages over other kinds of treatment for BPH. The procedure requires minimal or no hospitalization, and there's no need for a catheter following the implantation. That makes it an excellent choice for men who, for health reasons, may not be able to tolerate surgery or medical therapy. But there are also some drawbacks. Since the stent is a foreign body, no one knows how the body will respond to it over the long term. It irritates some men, at least initially—in clinical trials about 67 percent described urethral or bladder irritation for at least a month. In some cases it is bad enough that the stent must be removed.

The bottom line on stents is this: They are effective for a while in men who can't undergo surgery or take anti-BPH medications due to other health problems. They are also a good short-term alternative in men bothered by BPH symptoms who aren't expected to live many more years. But they are not currently a long-term solution for men suffering from a blocked urethra.

4

Understanding Prostate Cancer

The word *cancer* packs a tremendous emotional punch. In just six letters it spells fear, anger, pain, loss of control, and the specter of death. It is a disease that touches most of us, if not directly, then through a parent, a sibling, a child, friend, or coworker. Until recently, the statement "You have cancer" was akin to a death sentence. That's changing. Thanks to mammograms, blood tests, and a heightened awareness among Americans young and old, more and more cancers are being detected early while they're still curable.

Despite steady progress in the war against cancer, the number of people who succumb to the disease is likely to climb. Not because there's a "cancer epidemic," as popular magazines sometimes shout. The real culprit is modern medicine. Thanks to training and technology, physicians get better and better at detecting and diagnosing cancers—including prostate cancer—that once upon a time would have gone unnoticed. Modern medical care also keeps increasing numbers of people from dying in their fifties and early sixties of heart disease, diabetes, the complications of high blood pressure, and other chronic problems. Add to that the growing number of individuals who exercise, eat right, and don't smoke, and the result is a population that lives an average of seventy-five-plus years. So instead of dying young from a variety of diseases, more and more people are living to a ripe old age and dying from cancer, a disease to which aging clearly contributes.

What Is Cancer?

Perhaps the most insidious side of cancer is that it's a disease caused by your own cells turning against you. Bacterial and viral infections, food poisoning, snakebite—all make sense as health problems because they are threats from the hostile world beyond your skin. In a sense, the human body is a fortress designed to withstand threats from the outside world. Skin forms a mostly impenetrable layer; enzymes in tears kill bacteria; stomach acids and proteins destroy microbes that ride in on food. The immune system fights off invaders that breach these defenses. Cancer, however, starts out as a perfectly normal cell that turns renegade, subverting the body's defenses and even stealing its resources to grow, multiply, and sometimes kill.

Though cells from different body tissues look quite different, they actually share key similarities. All of the trillion or so cells in an individual's body are descended from the same ancestor, a single cell formed by the union of an egg and sperm. So they all have the same genetic makeup. A nerve cell, a white blood cell, and a liver cell from one person each contain the same set of forty-six chromosomes, faithful copies of the twenty-three pairs contained in the fertilized egg. Each chromosome is basically a string of genes, which are blueprints or instructions for particular cell functions.

If a lung cell and a skin cell have identical genes, how can they look and act so differently? As the early embryo divides into two cells, then four, eight, sixteen, thirty-two and so forth cells, each absorbing food, growing, and excreting wastes, small differences develop in the microenvironment around clusters of cells. One group responds to the tiny environmental difference by activating several genes. Another turns off certain genes, sometimes permanently.

Normal human cells are bound by a fairly strict code of conduct. They exhibit something called contact inhibition, meaning they won't continue to grow and divide when surrounded by other cells. Normal cells require nutrients such as sugar, amino acids, and vitamins plus special proteins called growth factors in order to survive and multiply. They resemble their parents—when a muscle cell divides into two daughter cells, the result is two muscle cells identical to the parent. And normal cells stay put, tightly connected to other, similar cells. Pancreas cells stay connected to the pancreas; they don't weigh anchor and drift through the bloodstream looking for a new home.

Cancer cells live by completely different rules. These turncoats happily grow one atop the other in great disorganized masses called tumors. They don't need the same carefully balanced cocktail of nutrients and growth factors as their normal counterparts. After several cell divisions, some cancer cells bear little resemblance to their recent ancestors. In fact, a kidney tumor may contain bits of bonelike tissue, or tissue that sprouts small hairs. Worst of all, cancer cells sometimes break away from the tumor, travel to a new part of the body, and put down roots. This process, called metastasis, is what makes cancer so deadly.

Once a tumor gets established, it doesn't grow passively, absorbing leftover nutrients. Instead, it aggressively reroutes the local blood flow by rearranging the plumbing. Tumor cells secrete proteins that stimulate the growth of new blood vessels. This trick ensures that nutrients will be delivered directly to the tumor—sometimes bypassing normal cells—and wastes will be removed.

How Cancer Spreads

If tumors were content to remain where they originated, cancer would be a far less deadly disease. So-called primary tumors account for only 10 percent of all cancer deaths, because they either aren't in a vital location or are too small to damage tissue. The real danger comes from metastasis, or cancer spreading through the body to a variety of different sites. A small tumor in the kidney may not disrupt kidney function. But breakaway cells that settle in the brain and interfere with the nerves that control breathing would have a major impact. Metastasis requires several complex steps, each of which reveals tumor cells as invidious and frighteningly well-adapted invaders.

Metastasis begins with one or more cells breaking away from the original tumor. If a cancer cell gets into the bloodstream, it can be carried far and wide throughout the body. Such free-ranging cells are commonly spotted by white blood cells and destroyed before they can leave the blood vessel. Occasionally, one either finds or creates a tiny break in the lining of a blood vessel. It then excavates a hole into the tissue below and burrows in. If this metastatic cell can draw enough nutrients to stay alive, it grows and divides, becoming the nucleus of a new tumor. Tumor cells can also find their way into the lymphatic system, a network of tiny vessels that collect and filter the fluids that bathe organs and tissues. In the lymphatic system, a cancer cell usually drifts to the first lymph node it encounters. If it manages to hide from white blood cells, it takes up residence in the node's maze of tiny filtration tubes and creates a new tumor.

No matter how a cancer cell gets from one place to another, the new tumor resembles the tissue in which it originated more than the one in which it resides. Prostate cancer that has metastasized to the pelvic bones, for example, does not become bonelike. It looks, acts, and secretes the same proteins as prostate tissue. In fact, it crowds out normal bone tissue, often weakening bones to the point where they spontaneously fracture.

Cancer is not a single disease like emphysema or insulin-dependent diabetes. Melanoma acts nothing like leukemia. Breast cancer behaves differently from bladder cancer. Each kind of cancer has its characteristic growth rate, preferred pattern of metastatic spread, and sensitivity to treatment. This diversity presents some difficulties for its victims and their physicians. Treatment that may obliterate one kind of tumor may have little impact on another. A breakthrough in detecting lung cancer won't necessarily translate to brain tumors. Prostate cancer's unique qualities make it both an easy and a difficult disease to deal with.

Prostate Cancer

Not too long ago, prostate cancer was considered just another old man's disease. It was rarely mentioned in public, received little attention in the media, and got scant funding for research. That's all changing. Today, prostate cancer is the most frequently diagnosed cancer in men; it passed lung cancer for this "honor" in 1992. The number of men diagnosed with the disease each year is increasing at a record pace, faster than for any other cancer since record keeping began. Stories on the disease regularly fill the pages of newspapers and magazines. The deaths of musician Frank Zappa and actors Bill Bixby and Telly Savalas thrust prostate cancer into the media spotlight. So too did the diagnosis and treatment of Senator Bob Dole of Kansas. Following his surgery in 1991, Dole has helped boost federal funding for prostate cancer research and has become a passionate spokesman on the disease. Before his speech at the 1992 Republican National Convention in Houston, for example, Dole urged the men over fifty in the audience and those watching on television to have yearly prostate exams. In 1994, legislators filed "The Prostate Cancer Diagnosis and Treatment Act" in the U.S. House and Senate to further stimulate federal research on this disease.

As cancers go, prostate cancer isn't the worst of the lot. Most early-stage prostate cancers are actually the slowest-growing cancers known, and they don't colonize other parts of the body as rapidly as lung, breast, or liver tumors do. In fact, the majority of men who have prostate cancer never realize it and die of a heart attack or old age instead. Simple tests can often detect an early-stage tumor long before it spreads to other parts of the body. And most tumors confined to the prostate that are detected early enough can be cured by surgery or radiation therapy.

The key phrase above is "early stage." Prostate cancer also has a dark, deadly side. Late-stage cancer that has spread beyond the prostate is generally not curable. Some men are afflicted with a fast-growing tumor that spreads rapidly to the bladder, bones, and other parts of the body. Such aggressive cancer can be reined in but never permanently stopped. It does not kill gently—men who die with metastatic prostate cancer often suffer excruciating pain that is difficult to control.

Today, there's really no way to tell the difference between a slow-growing prostate tumor and a virulent one. So men and their physicians generally approach a prostate tumor as they would an unfamiliar snake: assume it is dangerous until proven otherwise. This inability to distinguish relatively harmless from definitely deadly tumors is unfortunate, because the two main treatments for prostate cancer, surgery and radiation therapy, often leave behind long-term and potentially life-changing complications such as incontinence, impotence, rectal injury, and scarring of the urethra.

Tumor Growth

Like all cancers, prostate cancer starts out as a single cell dividing without restraint, unbound by the complex checks and balances that keep us from becoming disorganized masses of tissue. Assuming that this mutant cell and its offspring survive and escape detection by the immune system, they will eventually form a tumor. It takes about thirty rounds of cell division (one cell becomes two, two become four, four become eight . . .) to create the roughly 1 billion cells that make up a tumor one-half inch in diameter, the size of an acorn.

Approximately three-quarters of all prostate tumors originate inside the posterior portion of the prostate, the side that borders the rectum. That's why the rectal exam has traditionally been a valuable tool for spotting the disease. Using only a well-lubricated and gloved finger, a physician can digitally inspect much of the gland, prospecting for suspicious bumps or lumps. Normal prostate tissue feels firm but flexible, like the pad of the hand or tip of the nose. A cancerous prostate feels lumpy or knuckle hard. The digital exam cannot, however, pick up the 25 percent or so of tumors that grow deep inside the gland or on the surface facing away from the rectum.

A small, untreated tumor will grow and expand inside the gland. It gradually pushes out toward the surface of the prostate, works its way through the tough capsule, and emerges on the other side. Once the capsule has been breached, tumor cells almost invariably find their way to lymph nodes, bones, bladder, or other tissues. Sometimes cancer cells escape from the gland even before the capsule has been penetrated by working their way into blood or lymph vessels that run through the prostate and hitching a ride out. For some reason, prostate cancer cells often take up residence in bone tissue, especially the bones of the pelvis and spine. Perhaps bone marrow somehow protects these malignant cells from destruction by the immune system, or it offers them growth factors and other necessary nutrients not found elsewhere. In any case, tumors growing inside bony tissue eventually cause tough-to-treat pain. Other favorite sites for metastasizing prostate cancer cells are the bladder, lungs, liver, and lymph nodes in the pelvis.

With pancreatic or lung cancer, progression from small tumor to large tumor occurs very fast, and metastases can spread like wildfire. That's not necessarily the case for prostate cancer. As mentioned earlier, this is usually a very slow-growing cancer. Whereas a lung tumor may double in size in as little as three months, a nonaggressive prostate tumor takes three to four years. That means it may take nine to twelve years for a pinhead-sized tumor totally confined to the prostate gland to become a marble-sized one growing into or through the capsule. This slow growth pattern also explains why prostate cancer can recur ten to fifteen years after what appeared to have been successful treatment. It can take that long for a micro-scopic clump of cells that had escaped the gland before treatment to grow to a harmful size.

If all prostate cancers grew slowly, they would be much easier to treat. They don't. Some are tortoises, growing slowly for a very long time and then turning aggressive. Others are hares right away, starting as fast-growing cells and getting more virulent as they develop. Unfortunately, no tests accurately predict what a given tumor will do. Two come close. The Gleason grading scale and ploidy tests, which measure how many sets of chromosomes the average cancer cell contains, help predict whether a partic-ular tumor is a tortoise or a hare. Both are described in Chapter 6.

Diagnosis

The American Cancer society estimates that 240,000 men will be diagnosed with prostate cancer in 1995, and 40,000 will die from it. Put another way, every two min-utes another man learns he has the disease; every thirteen minutes someone dies of it—110 deaths each day from this disease.

These numbers are actually just the tip of the iceberg. Autopsies of men who have died suddenly—in auto acci-dents, of violence, of heart attacks, etc.—show that 20 percent of men in their fifties have microscopic evidence of prostate cancer. This rises to 40 percent of men in their seventies and half or more of all men eighty and older. Applying these estimates to the current U.S. population suggests that roughly 11 million men are walking around today with a tiny cluster of cancer cells in their prostates. These cells generally divide so slowly that the vast majority of prostate tumors never grow large enough to be noticed by a man or his physician, even those who do the most careful rectal exams. Nor will they cause any symptoms or shorten lives. Only about 10 percent ever develop into full-blown prostate cancer; and only 3 percent cause death.

These grim statistics hide some encouraging news about the disease. The rapid increase in cases diagnosed each year is testimony to a growing awareness of the disease. More and more men are asking their physicians to check their prostates and perform a relatively new test called the prostate-specific antigen test, or PSA. This simple, relatively inexpensive blood test can often detect tumors too small to raise a bump on the prostate. At this point, the chance of a complete cure is quite high. The odds that a well-differentiated tumor smaller than a marble has spread beyond the gland are only five in 100. Most men treated for tumors this size live out their normal lives and die of something other than prostate cancer. Once a tumor has grown through the gland's capsule and spread beyond it, the likelihood of a cure dwindles.

Before the PSA test came into widespread use in the late 1980s, between half and two-thirds of men diagnosed with prostate cancer were initially diagnosed with advanced prostate cancer. Today, that's down to almost one quarter. Or, put more positively, today almost 75 percent of men discover their prostate cancer while it is still theoretically curable. The lone drawback of the PSA test is that it sometimes detects small prostate tumors that would never have affected a man's health or long life. Since detection usually leads to treatment, and treatment can mean potentially life-changing side effects, a vigorous debate is brewing among researchers and physicians about PSA screening.

Most men have no inkling they have prostate cancer. Since it rarely announces its presence with definable symptoms, it usually comes as a great surprise. Symptoms usually appear only after a tumor has grown to a substantial size in the gland or has spread beyond it. Even then, symptoms aren't clear-cut; many are blamed on getting older or confused with other ailments. The most common ones include:

- A noticeable weakening of the urine stream, or difficulty starting and stopping urination, caused by a tumor pressing on the urethra. Each of these is commonly associated with aging, and also occurs, because of benign prostate enlargement or infection of the gland.
- Nagging low-back pain often extending into the pelvic region, buttocks, or thighs, usually caused by metastatic tumors growing in the bones and pressing on nerves. Such pains can also come from arthritis, "a bad back," or degenerative disk disease.
- Constipation, which sometimes occurs when a prostate tumor grows large enough to press into the rectum. Poor diet, many medications, and old age all cause constipation.
- Weight loss, which often accompanies many cancers. Again, poor diet, medications, depression, and a host of diseases cause men to lose weight.

- Loss of erections sometimes results when a prostate tumor interferes with the nerves or blood vessels that control erectile function. Impotence is a complex problem, sparked sometimes by emotional or psychological factors, and sometimes by physical factors. These include poor circulation, heart disease, smoking, and many medications.

Causes and Risk Factors

Prostate cancer has several clear risk factors, most of which a man can't control—age, functioning testicles, race, and genetics. A few external factors, however, may also play a role. Working with cadmium, a metal used in batteries and electroplating, may make a man slightly more prone to developing prostate cancer. And a high-fat, low-fiber diet also appears to predispose one to the disease.

Age

The older a man gets, the more likely he is to be diagnosed with prostate cancer. The statistic mentioned most frequently in news reports and magazine articles is that U.S. males have a one in ten lifetime chance of being diagnosed with the disease. That doesn't mean one member of your softball team is sure to get prostate cancer, because such statistics only apply to large groups of men and even then only when spread over a lifetime.

The table in figure 4.1 tells the story a bit more clearly. It lists the odds that men of different ages will be diagnosed with prostate cancer. In 1994, men ages forty to forty-four faced a one in 48,640 chance of hearing a

Figure 4.1. Odds of being diagnosed with prostate cancer

Age	Odds of diagnosis
20–39	insignificant
40–44	1 in 48,640
45–49	1 in 9,085
50–54	1 in 1,943
55–59	1 in 624
60–64	1 in 240
65–69	1 in 122
70–74	1 in 81
75–79	1 in 65
80–84	1 in 58
85+	1 in 63

SOURCES: number of cancer cases by age from the American Cancer Society; number of men by age from the U.S. Bureau of the Census.

physician tell them they have prostate cancer. For men forty-five to forty-nine the odds rose to one in 9,085. (Even at those odds, approximately 1,100 men under fifty were diagnosed with prostate cancer in 1994.) By age seventy-five, a man stands a one in sixty-five chance of being diagnosed with prostate cancer. Why age plays such a role in prostate cancer isn't clear. Perhaps the tumors grow so slowly in most men that it takes several decades for them to pose a medical problem. Or perhaps the longer a man lives, the more likely he is to be exposed to some as-yet-undiscovered risk factor. It may also take years for prostate cells to accumulate the two genetic hits needed to trigger cancer.

The words "old" and "young" take on new meaning when used in the context of prostate cancer. Anyone under sixty diagnosed with this disease is "young," and "old" usually refers to men over seventy-five. "That was the one good thing about having prostate cancer," says Eddie, a fifty-nine-year-old truck driver. "Everyone kept referring to me as a young man."

Hormones

One clear prerequisite for the development of prostate cancer is functioning testicles. Men who were castrated early in life, or those whose testes were irreparably damaged, rarely, if ever, fall victim to this disease. Without working testes a man can't manufacture testosterone, the male hormone that signals both normal and malignant prostate cells to grow and divide. With functioning testes he can. (This connection formed the basis for hormone therapy, widely used to treat advanced prostate cancer. See Chapter 10.) You might think, then, that men who have low levels of circulating testosterone would be less likely to develop prostate cancer and those who have high levels are more prone to it. In fact, research hasn't supported such a relationship.

Country and Race

Prostate cancer is not an equal-opportunity disease. Japanese and Chinese men are the least likely to die from it. At the other end of the spectrum, African-American men have the highest incidence of prostate cancer in the world. Geography, nationality, and culture somehow influence the development of this disease. The incidence is lowest in the Orient and increases across Europe, peaking in Scandinavia and Switzerland. Only a few explanations have been offered for this trend. Some researchers think that diet may be involved. An intriguing study from the University of North Carolina pointed out that higher rates of prostate cancer often appear in regions of less sunlight where people's bodies tend to manufacture less vitamin D. Dark skin may also reduce the synthesis of vitamin D, which could explain why black men have higher rates of prostate cancer than white men.

The United States falls in the upper end of the spectrum, with prostate cancer striking approximately ninety per 100,000 men. This average disguises a sharp racial difference—black Americans are diagnosed with prostate cancer at a rate of 120 per 100,000 men, while for white Americans the rate is only 75 per 100,000. Death rates show an even more marked difference.

Black men also are initially diagnosed with metastatic prostate cancer more frequently than white men. This can be partially explained by socioeconomic status and the fact that blacks generally have less access to health care than whites in the United States. But there's more to it than that. In a study of a new therapy for prostate cancer, black men died an average of six months sooner than white men with the same-stage tumor. Another study compared young black men and young white men diagnosed with early-onset prostate cancer who received identical treatment. The black men lived an average of 3.9 years, the white men 6.0 years.

Family History

Physicians have long suspected that prostate cancer runs in families. That's certainly the case for breast cancer—having a mother or sister with breast cancer doubles a woman's chance of developing the disease. However, inherited "bad genes" probably aren't responsible for the bulk of prostate cancer, especially in older men. That two eightysomething brothers have prostate cancer may be more coincidence than a defective gene, given the high odds for this disease at that age.

But an inherited gene may be responsible for prostate tumors that appear early, before age sixty. Researchers at the Johns Hopkins Medical Institutions in Baltimore compared 690 men with early prostate cancer to a similar number without it. They found that a man whose father or brother was diagnosed with prostate cancer was twice as likely to develop the disease as a man with no affected relatives. Having a father and two brothers afflicted with the disease increases the risk elevenfold (fig. 4.2).

All men can apply this important discovery to their own lives. If you vaguely recall that someone in your extended family has had prostate cancer, make a few phone calls to your close relatives. Gather enough information to make a simple family tree (fig. 4.3). Include relatives on both your mother's and father's side—grandparents, uncles, brothers, nephews. (There's no need to include your sister's hus-

Figure 4.2. Relative risk of developing prostate cancer for relatives

NUMBER OF AFFECTED RELATIVES	RELATIVE RISK
Father and/or brothers	
One	Twofold
Two	Fivefold
Three or more	11-fold
Father/brother or grandfather/uncle	
One	1.5-fold
Two	2.3-fold
Three or more	3.6-fold

SOURCE: Dr. Patrick C. Walsh, Johns Hopkins Hospital. Used with permission.

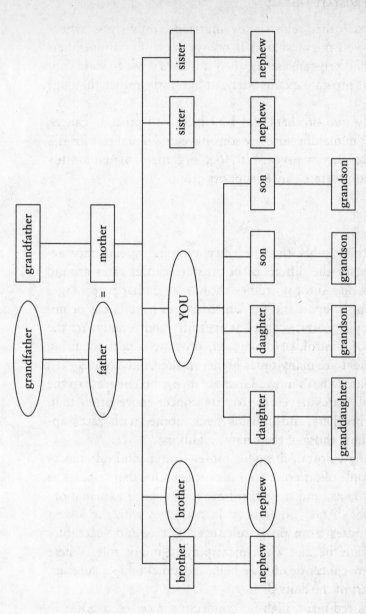

Figure 4.3. Constructing a Family Tree. By circling the male family members known to have or have had prostate cancer, one can get an idea as to whether the disease is inherited in your family. Inheritance is suggested if there is a pattern rather than a random occurrence. In this example, a pattern of inheritance is shown suggesting that in this family cancer of the prostate is inherited. The males in the fourth and fifth generations are at higher risk and should be more vigilant about checkups.

band or other relatives by marriage; only those whose genes you might share.) If one or more family members have had prostate cancer, then it makes sense to start your annual prostate exams early, at age forty rather than age fifty.

"My two brothers and I all have had prostate cancer. Now I'm making sure my sons have an annual test for it," says seventy-two-year-old Joe, organizer of a monthly Us-Too prostate cancer support group.

Diet

Something other than heredity, nationality, and race accounts for the difference in prostate cancer rates around the world. Autopsy studies show that similar percentages of men in Japan and the United States have latent or microscopic prostate cancer at ages fifty and seventy. Yet the rates of clinical, or diagnosed, prostate cancer requiring treatment are many times higher in the United States than in Japan. What's more, Japanese men who emigrate to the United States develop prostate cancer more often than their brothers and cousins back home, with rates approaching those of their new neighbors.

Many cultural, lifestyle, and environmental differences set people of different countries apart. One that appears to fit the facts, and may also have a biological explanation, involves dietary differences. In countries with the lowest death rates from prostate cancer, grains and vegetables dominate the diet while meat plays a minor role. Where prostate cancer deaths are high, meat makes up a substantial part of the daily diet.

This red-meat, high-fat connection received a boost in 1993 from a long-term study of 59,000 male health-care professionals. Two Harvard researchers found that the men in the study who ate five or more meal-sized portions of red meat a week developed advanced prostate cancer 2.6 times more often than those who ate meat once a week or less. One suspect may be a saturated fat called alpha-linolenic acid found in red meat. Cells need a minuscule amount of this substance for normal growth and cell division. Feeding precancerous cells too much alpha-linolenic acid might kick them into overdrive. The researchers found *no* association between high animal fat intake and early-stage prostate cancer. This could mean that dietary fat doesn't initiate tumor growth—make the first genetic hit—but instead may push normal-acting cells that contain a genetic mistake or two over the edge toward malignancy.

Diet may play a role in other ways. Several studies in the United States and elsewhere show that men who eat foods high in fiber (bran, oatmeal, fresh fruits and vegetables) are less likely to develop prostate cancer than the average U.S. male. Fiber, it turns out, may lower the amount of estrogen and testosterone circulating in the blood. As fiber passes through the intestines, it appears to absorb hormones, much like a sponge soaking up spilled water. When the fiber exits the body in the stool, it carries along a dose of sex hormones. Since testosterone stimulates the growth of prostate-cancer cells, hormone-eliminating fiber could lower the risk.

A study of 14,000 Seventh-Day Adventist men also revealed an interesting connection between diet and cancer: increasing the weekly consumption of peas, tomatoes, beans, and raisins and other dried fruit appears to protect against prostate cancer. All are low-fat, high-fiber foods and thus may work as described above. They may also contribute trace minerals or vitamins that somehow protect against prostate cancer.

A host of studies from reputable cancer researchers

across the country suggest that diet plays an important role in abetting or preventing breast, colon, stomach, and other cancers. While the mechanism isn't clear, it may involve natural cancer-fighting compounds that have been discovered in foods like broccoli and celery. Based on this mounting body of evidence, the National Cancer Institute has begun educating the American public about yet another benefit of eating right. Its "Five Alive" campaign recommends that a healthy diet may help prevent certain cancers from developing. The NCI defines healthy as low-fat, high-fiber, and including at least five servings of fresh fruit and vegetables a day.

Such a diet is no guarantee against prostate cancer. Even strict vegetarians who exercise regularly, don't smoke or drink, and work in the great outdoors get prostate cancer. So beware of claims promoting miracle diets, foods, or supplements guaranteed to prevent prostate cancer. Several "anti-prostate-cancer supplements" are available in health-food stores and alternative pharmacies. No hard evidence exists that any of these work. Some are merely an expensive way of taking the same nutrients you could get by eating an extra piece of fruit a day. Others could actually be hazardous to your health, especially if taken in too large a quantity or with some medications.

Sexual Activity

At one point, prostate cancer and benign prostatic hyperplasia were said to arise when too little sexual activity caused congestion of the prostate. Dozens of recent data-laden studies on the sex-cancer association have failed to come up with clear answers. Frequent or infrequent ejaculations, having sex with many partners, infection with a sexually transmitted disease, masturbation, early or late first sexual experience—none appears to raise or lower a man's chance of developing prostate cancer.

A 1992 study earned national headlines for describing an apparent connection between prostate cancer and vasectomy, a popular operation that renders a man infertile. Men with the operation, the researchers found, were 2.9 times more likely to be diagnosed with prostate cancer than men of similar ages and socioeconomic levels who had never had the operation. At a quickly convened conference sponsored by the National Cancer Institute and American Urological Association, cancer experts concluded that vasectomy probably does not *cause* prostate cancer. Instead, the men who choose this method of birth control may have more frequent medical checkups than the average man. And more checkups mean more chances to detect a prostate lump or nodule.

Smoking

This shouldn't come as a surprise: Smoking probably increases your chances of developing prostate cancer. The link isn't as ironclad as the cigarette–lung cancer connection. But a handful of large studies from several countries suggest that men who smoke are more likely to end up with prostate cancer than men who don't. On top of that, men who smoke are more likely to become impotent following treatment for prostate cancer, and generally recover from procedures more slowly.

Steroids

Once limited to the shady side of professional sports, steroid use has spilled over into community weight rooms and high-school locker rooms. These synthetic hormones offer men a relatively quick way to add muscle. Anabolic steroids basically mimic testosterone's muscle-building effects. They speed recovery after strenuous exercise and thus allow a more demanding training schedule. Many men, however, pay a price for these instant muscles. Steroid abuse causes acne, damages the liver and adrenal glands, and can lead to impotence or infertility. Now it appears that the testosterone-like activity of these drugs may stimulate the growth of prostate and prostate-cancer cells. Physicians around the country have begun reporting cases of early-onset prostate cancer in men who routinely used steroids. While there's not yet enough data to pin down this association, men who use or have used anabolic steroids may want to be especially diligent about annual prostate cancer checkups and may also want to begin them at age forty rather than age fifty.

Occupation

Men working in every industry and at every occupation get prostate cancer. (The only exception might have been castrated men charged with guarding the sultans' harems!) A number of very small, very preliminary studies have suggested that several occupations or industries—plumbers, farmers, mechanics, newspaper workers, or men working in rubber manufacturing plants—may be associated with higher-than-expected rates of this disease. None of these reports has been confirmed.

As mentioned earlier, one occupational exposure does seem to merit some attention. Men who work with cadmium seem to develop prostate cancer more than other men. Cadmium is a metal used in batteries and the electroplating industry. Some preliminary studies suggest that prolonged exposure to it may slightly increase a man's chances of being diagnosed with a prostate tumor.

5

Preventing
Prostate Cancer

If you stop smoking, you dramatically reduce your chances of developing lung cancer. To limit your risk of getting skin cancer, don't get sunburned or bake yourself in the sun. Unfortunately, there's no simple prescription for preventing prostate cancer. That's because no one knows exactly what causes this common disease. There is no changing the two leading risk factors—you can't pull a Dorian Gray and stop aging, nor do you want to live without functioning testes. Changing your race or the genes you inherited from your parents aren't options. What you *can* do is watch your diet, have regular physical exams that include a rectal exam and PSA test, and follow what most of us would call a healthy lifestyle—don't smoke, drink in moderation, and exercise regularly. And if you're feeling public spirited, you might join an ongoing clinical trial designed to see if daily doses of a chemical called finasteride ward off prostate cancer.

Eating Right

As mentioned in Chapter 4, a high-fat, low-fiber diet somehow leads men down the road to prostate disease. Something about that kind of food either damages normal prostate cells and pushes them toward malignancy or encourages already-damaged cells to ignore the normal signals that limit cell growth and division. This diet connection isn't unique to prostate cancer. Women who eat a high-fat, low-fiber diet are more prone to developing breast cancer, and colon cancer seems to strike more often in individuals who follow this kind of diet.

The National Cancer Institute (NCI) has published guidelines for a healthy diet that rates high on the cancer-prevention scale. Most of your daily calories should come from carbohydrates and protein, with only 30 percent or less coming from fats. Whenever possible, stay away from saturated fats—solid or congealable fats such as those found in meat and dairy products. No one knows the precise mechanism that links fat to prostate cancer, though researchers suspect it may be a saturated-fat component called alpha-linolenic acid. Small doses of this substance stimulate cell growth and division, so the large daily doses that come with a meat-heavy diet may really rev up this process.

Following the NCI's advice doesn't condemn you to a life of sprouts and tofu burgers. Eat chicken and fish more often, and limit your steaks and barbecued ribs to special occasions.

Fiber and natural vitamins are also important components of a healthy diet. As fiber passes through your intestines, it acts like a scouring brush that pushes food and potentially toxic chemicals through more quickly. It may also absorb hormones and hormone-like substances, especially the kind that stimulate prostate cancer growth. Vitamins and other plant compounds are also crucial. A variety of chemicals found in broccoli, celery, and other foods may actually fight cancer. Antioxidant compounds found in a wide range of fruits and vegetables may detoxify pesticide residues, cooking by-products, and other potentially cancer-causing chemicals you take in with your food.

While vitamin manufacturers tout the value of their products, what you get from a bottle just isn't the same as what you get from fresh, frozen, or dried fruits and vegetables. Granted, the vitamin C you get in a vitamin tablet is chemically identical to the vitamin C in a glass of orange juice. Both are absorbed by the body and perform the same tasks. But all you get from the tablet is vitamin C, while the glass of juice contains dozens of other compounds that may either enhance its activity or offer even greater benefits.

For this reason the NCI also recommends five servings of fresh fruits or vegetables a day. That amounts to a glass of fresh juice and a banana with cereal for breakfast, an apple with lunch, and a potato and green beans with dinner. Throw in a salad—hold the Caesar dressing—and you're really in business.

Should You Think Zinc?

You may have read that the mineral zinc can prevent prostate cancer. Such reports are more confusion or wishful thinking than reality. Here are the hard facts: A normal, healthy prostate gland contains higher levels of zinc than any other body tissue. Men with prostate cancer often have lower than normal amounts of zinc inside the gland or its fluids. But no one knows if low zinc levels *cause* prostate cancer or if prostate cancer somehow makes the gland lose zinc. Furthermore, clinical and laboratory studies suggest the prostate gland may not be able to absorb the kind of zinc found in vitamin pills or supplements from the bloodstream. If you want to give yourself a zinc boost, add these foods to your diet: pumpkin seeds, lentils, liver, chicken, wheat germ, oysters, and peas.

Steroids and Smoking

In addition to eating right, here are two activities to avoid if you wish to ward off prostate cancer:

• Don't fool around with anabolic steroids to build muscle. These compounds may act like fertilizer for prostate and prostate-cancer cells. If you've used them in the past, you might want to start your annual prostate checkups at age forty or forty-five instead of age fifty.

• Don't smoke. Not only does this habit predispose you to a variety of other cancers as well as prostate cancer, it also makes you a more likely candidate for complications if you're ever treated for cancer.

Joining a Chemoprevention Trial

Across the United States, thousands of men take a tablet of the drug finasteride (Proscar) every day. This substance, recently approved as a treatment for benign prostatic hyperplasia, halts the conversion of testosterone into its even-more-active cousin, 5-dihydrotestosterone (5-DHT) inside the prostate gland. Without sufficient 5-DHT, prostate cells grow and divide even more slowly than usual. And if it can do that for normal cells, researchers reason, then it may have the same effect on prostate-cancer cells or those with a precancerous attitude. Thus was born the Prostate Cancer Prevention Trial, an ambitious effort to find a way to prevent prostate cancer.

Finasteride is an attractive drug for this effort. It is known to slow the growth of prostate cells. Even more valuable, it acts only on tissues that convert testosterone to 5-DHT. That means it affects a limited number of organs—basically the prostate and testes—and has no effect on the heart, liver, brain, or other systems. Such specific activity leads to a narrow spectrum of side effects. In the clinical trials sponsored by Merck and Company, Proscar's manufacturer, more than one thousand men with BPH took the drug or a placebo, a pill made of sugar or other innocuous substance, for months. Decreased sexual desire was reported by 3.3 percent of men who took finasteride, compared with 1.6 percent of men given a placebo; 3.7 percent of those taking finasteride had some difficulty with erections, while 1.1 percent of the placebo group had the same problem; and 2.8 percent of the finasteride group said the amount of fluid they ejaculated was less than normal, while only 0.9 percent of those taking the placebo said this.

A recent study suggests that these side effects tend to disappear as men take the drug for longer periods. However, since finasteride has only been available for a few years, there are virtually no data on whether long-term use has any surprising consequences.

To accurately measure finasteride's effects, researchers need to enroll 18,000 men into the Prostate Cancer Prevention Trial. All will take a small pill every day for seven years, but only half will actually be taking finasteride. The others will take an identical placebo. Neither the men, their physicians, nor the researchers running the trial will know who is taking what until it's time to analyze the outcomes in about ten years. This is what's called a "double-blind" trial, the gold standard in research. Although use of the placebo pill may seem deceptive, it's a crucial part of the trial. Without it, researchers would have no way to tell if finasteride makes a difference.

Any man fifty-five or older who is in good health and free of prostate cancer can enroll in the trial. All participants receive their finasteride (or placebo) free. They also get free annual PSA tests as well as a prostate biopsy at the end of seven years. The only thing the participants pay for is their own routine medical care, which must include an annual physical that includes a rectal exam. A call to the National Cancer Institute at 800-4-CANCER is all it takes to get directions to the nearest medical center participating in the trial.

6

Making the Diagnosis

For the majority of men, the diagnosis of prostate cancer arrives suddenly and unexpectedly, like a lightning bolt and the clap of rumbling thunder that follows. A few men have an inkling that something is wrong because of odd, unexplained pains or trouble urinating.

Bernie, a sixty-four-year-old investment counselor, started down the road to diagnosis one morning when he had to rush to an emergency room, completely unable to empty his overfull bladder. Seventy-six-year-old Joseph went to his physician several times complaining of persistent lower-back pain before discovering that advanced prostate cancer was the cause. Justin, a seventy-year-old dentist, had put off having a complete physical exam for years, mostly because he wasn't wild about the idea of a digital rectal exam. His physician finally talked him into it, and found nothing; but a special blood test came back above normal. Sixty-eight-year-old John, a retired public-relations executive, had a series of checkups after he began to have trouble urinating. On the sixth or seventh visit to a physician, his doctor told him he "might have a little problem." It turned out to be a malignant lump. Bill, a sixty-six-year-old former lighting engineer, didn't suspect a thing when he walked into a local hospital's free screening during Prostate Awareness Week. He walked out a bit worried and, once the results of his blood test were in, with good reason.

This disease isn't as easy to diagnose as pneumonia, say, or high blood pressure. Most prostate tumors grow for years without generating any warning signals. And when symptoms do appear, they are easily mistaken for the signs of old age or other diseases. To make matters worse, no single test short of removing and inspecting the gland can say with absolute certainty that you have prostate cancer. For these reasons, a man whose physician suspects this disease can expect to face a battery of tests designed to accomplish different crucial tasks:

- Rule out other diseases such as benign prostatic hyperplasia, prostate infection, or bladder disease.
- Measure the size and location of a suspected tumor and estimate if it is confined to the gland or has spread beyond it.
- Predict whether a tumor, if present, is of the slow-growing or fast-spreading type.

The diagnostic tests described on the following pages are those a man is most likely to encounter. The first three—rectal exam, blood and urine tests, and biopsy—are the standards. The others may be needed if the tumor is a large one or may have spread outside the prostate.

Digital Rectal Exam

This simple, quick, inexpensive test has been the mainstay of prostate cancer detection for almost a century. I include a rectal exam as part of a general checkup for my male patients since it can also spot early colon or rectal cancer. For several seconds of very mild discomfort and no side effects, it offers tremendous benefits. Unfortunately, half or more of primary-care physicians forgo this simple but crucial test, according to an American Cancer Society survey. That translates into this tragic statistic—up to 70 percent of men over fifty don't get a rectal exam each year. If your physician finishes a physical exam without doing this test, *ask* him or her to do it. It can save your life.

The digital rectal exam begins with you either lying on your side on an examining table, knees drawn up, or bending over the table. In either case, your physician will insert a gloved, well-lubricated finger into your rectum. The natural response is to tighten the sphincter at the first touch, even though relaxing will make it easier for both of you. It's also perfectly normal to feel as though you need to defecate during the exam. Don't worry, you won't.

With a finger inside the rectum, your physician can feel the prostate through the rectal wall. He or she uses a side-to-side sweeping motion to cover as much of the gland as possible. Checking for a deep-seated tumor may require a gentle press or two. Some men find the ten-second procedure totally innocuous. Others say it is literally a pain in the rear.

A perfectly healthy prostate feels smooth, firm, and a bit rubbery to the touch, much like the tip of the nose. So physicians let their fingers look for any irregularities like a bump or hard patch on the prostate. Not finding one is a good sign, but it's no guarantee that the gland is cancer-free. Tumors can live deep inside the gland and not raise a lump on the surface. And about 20 percent of all prostate tumors grow on the side of the prostate away from the rectum, where a physician's finger can't reach. A rectal exam can also turn up other problems such as colon cancer, hemorrhoids, and prostate infection. This versatility makes it an essential part of a man's general medical exam.

PSA Test

Some of the tumors missed by a rectal exam can be detected by a relatively new blood test. The PSA—short for prostate-specific antigen—test measures the blood levels of a protein manufactured by prostate cells. While it is fairly effective at detecting cancer all by itself, several studies have shown that the most effective combination for finding prostate cancer is PSA plus a digital rectal exam.

The exact physiological role of prostate-specific antigen isn't known. Made by a special gland in the prostate, it is propelled into the urethra at ejaculation. There it mixes with semen, either to keep seminal fluid from coagulating or to break up tiny clots of semen that lodge in the reproductive tract or urethra. Normally, very little PSA gets into the bloodstream. But benign prostatic hyperplasia, prostate infection, or a tumor can break tiny blood vessels or make prostate cells "leaky." In each case this protein drips into the circulation and elevates a man's PSA level.

After prostate-specific antigen was discovered in the early 1970s, forensic scientists devised a test for the protein. Since prostate secretions contain PSA, the test became widely used for determining if a fluid or stain found at a crime scene contained semen. Techniques developed in the mid-1980s allowed laboratories to measure the *amount* of this protein in a blood sample. This gave physicians a powerful way to indirectly track the growth of prostate cells without inspecting the gland. The higher the PSA, the more prostate and prostate-cancer cells present in the body.

For the most commonly used PSA test, normal is considered anything below 4.0. PSA numbers refer to nanograms of protein per milliliter of blood. (A nanogram is a billionth of a gram; a milliliter a thousandth of a liter. A nanogram per milliliter is the equivalent of tossing a cup of protein into a container of water the size of the *Exxon Valdez*.) Some physicians think a sliding scale might be more accurate, since older men tend to secrete more PSA even in the absence of prostate cancer. One such age-specific scale sets 2.5 as the upper limit for normal in men forty to forty-nine; 3.5 for men fifty to fifty-nine; 4.5 for men sixty to sixty-nine; and 6.5 for men over seventy. This scale could increase the number of cancers detected early in younger men but may miss some cancers in older men.

Keep in mind that the PSA test is not a true diagnostic test. A pregnancy test, for example, tells a woman she either is or isn't pregnant. The PSA, by comparison, can only suggest the possibility of cancer. There are several reasons for this:

• *All* prostate cells produce prostate-specific antigen. A man with a naturally large prostate or with benign prostatic hyperplasia (noncancerous prostate enlargement) will generally have an above-normal PSA level. As many as 70 percent of all men with a PSA between 4.0 and 10.0 *do not have prostate cancer.*

• Not all men with prostate cancer have above-normal PSA levels. Between 25 percent and 45 percent of men ultimately found to have prostate cancer by other tests have PSA readings below 4.0.

• An unnoticed prostate infection can elevate PSA levels above normal. So can excessive pressure on the gland, such as that caused by a transurethral resection of the prostate, cystoscopy, or other procedure which squeezes the gland and expels stored fluid from it. (Neither a digital rectal exam nor sexual activity just prior to the test significantly influences the results.)

Because of these conditions, it's wise to be a tad skeptical of a single PSA reading. If your first-ever PSA is normal and your physician didn't find any suspicious bumps on your prostate, great. But don't take that news as a clean bill of health for the next decade or so. Mark your calendar for another prostate checkup in a year to make sure that a new tumor hasn't appeared or a previously hidden one hasn't emerged. As mentioned earlier, these tumors generally grow slowly, so once-a-year checkups are plenty.

If the test comes back above normal, your physician will probably have it repeated to make sure the results were accurate. If they are, he or she will suggest you have a transrectal ultrasound-guided biopsy (see page 99) and perhaps several additional tests.

Attempts at improving PSA-type tests are currently under way. One from Memorial–Sloan Kettering Cancer Center in New York uses an antibody to find cells that make prostate-specific-membrane antigen, a protein found on the exterior of prostate and prostate-cancer cells. Preliminary studies suggest that this test could detect prostate tumors that don't make excess PSA. Another one under development here at the Massachusetts General Hospital and elsewhere finds PSA-making cells that have broken away from the prostate and are circulating in the bloodstream. With such a test in hand, clinicians could more accurately identify when a tumor has spread outside the prostate gland and make more accurate decisions about treatment. Further study is needed, however.

Another refinement entails separating free PSA from PSA bound to carrier proteins. It appears that men with prostate cancer have a higher percentage of bound PSA than men with BPH or men with perfectly normal prostates.

Other Laboratory Tests

At the same time blood is drawn for your PSA, vials will also be taken for other tests. A laboratory technician will count the number of red and white cells per milliliter of blood, to make sure no infection or other imbalance is present that might mimic the signs of prostate cancer. Other standard tests:

• *Acid phosphatase* is another protein made by prostate and prostate cancer cells. An above-normal pros-tatic-acid-phosphatase reading suggests that a tumor may have spread beyond the prostate. Together with a bone scan (see page 105) it can be helpful in identifying metastatic disease.

• *Serum creatinine* measures kidney function. Creatinine is a waste product normally excreted in urine; above-normal levels indicate kidney distress possibly caused by a tumor blocking urine flow.

- *Evaluation of a urine sample* can rule out prostate or urinary-tract infection as the reason for urinary symptoms or an elevated PSA. No needles are involved—you merely wash your hands and the head of your penis with antiseptic soap and then urinate into a sterile plastic cup. Bacteria, sediment, or white blood cells in the urine suggest an infection that can usually be treated with antibiotics (see Chapter 2). The presence of red blood cells, which normally aren't found in the urine, suggests that something else—benign hyperplasia or a tumor—is disrupting the normal gland structure and blood flow.

Transrectal Ultrasound

If a rectal exam or PSA test indicates a tumor may be present, ultrasound can help refine the diagnosis. As its name implies, this test uses sound waves to map the prostate, bladder, and surrounding structures and to reveal a tumor's size and location. Ultrasound is a commonly used diagnostic tool. Its other uses include checking on fetuses months before they are born, looking for pelvic masses or kidney dysfunction, and examining arteries for accumulated cholesterol-laden plaque.

The test works just like the sonar systems you've seen in countless World War II submarine-versus-destroyer movies on television. Sound waves pitched far above what our ears can hear are fired at the prostate. Some are absorbed, some bounce off at an angle, others bounce back to a receiver. The waves travel at different speeds through different tissues—faster in dense tissue, slower in loose tissue. (Sound travels faster in water than air because water molecules are closer together and pass along vibrations more readily.) A computer takes the jumble of reflected sound waves and organizes it into a coherent landscape (fig. 6.1).

The night before an ultrasound you'll be asked to take some antibiotics and give yourself an enema to clean out the rectum and colon. The scan itself takes about five to ten minutes. It uses a miniaturized sound-wave generator and receiver packed into a sausage-shaped tube and connected to a computer (fig. 6.2). As you lie on your back or side on an examination table, knees up, the lubricated ultrasound probe is inserted into your rectum. As with the rectal exam, you may feel some discomfort. The sensation that you need to defecate is also entirely normal. You won't feel or hear the ultrasound waves bouncing around your prostate as the physician or technician positions the

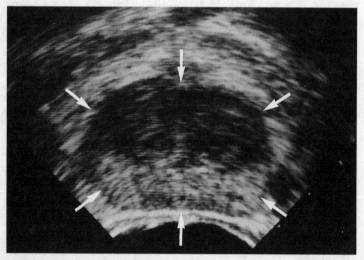

Figure 6.1. *An ultrasound of a normal prostate. The arrows highlight the gland's outline.*

probe to get the clearest image possible. Once that's accomplished, he or she will snap a few pictures and remove the probe.

A normal prostate has the same density throughout, which appears as a single shade of gray on the monitor or in photos. Tumors are more or less dense than healthy tissue, and so appear as lighter or darker spots.

Biopsy

While transrectal ultrasound is sometimes used to find a tumor, it plays an even more important role in guiding a biopsy, or tissue sample. The biopsy is perhaps the ultimate test for prostate cancer short of removing and inspecting the entire gland. Until recently, a biopsy took

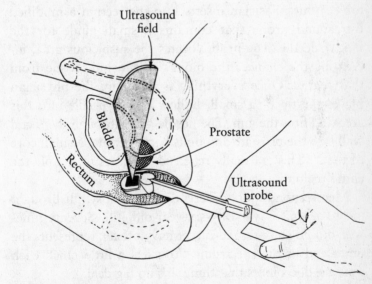

Figure 6.2. *The ultrasound probe is inserted into the rectum and positioned immediately below the prostate.*

almost that much work. To get a sample of prostate tissue, a surgeon once had to operate, with the patient under general anesthesia. Through an incision between the anus and scrotum, he or she would find the prostate under layers of other tissue, take a slice or two near where the suspected tumor resided, and then close up the incision. This major surgery required a several-day hospital stay, and was done when a suspicious nodule couldn't be identified as cancerous or benign. The advent of spring-loaded biopsy "guns" made the procedure far simpler and safer, but not much different from shooting in the dark.

Today, thanks to transrectal ultrasound and biopsy guns, the procedure can be completed in several minutes in a physician's office. For you, the procedure is almost identical to having a plain transrectal ultrasound. You lie on your back or side, knees drawn up, on an examination table. Your physician inserts into the rectum a modified ultrasound probe that contains a small guide for the biopsy needle. The probe locates the suspicious area, increasing the chances the biopsy will include tissue from that region. Once everything is lined up, the physician places the tip of a small, hollow biopsy needle into this area and fires the gun. The needle darts through the rectal wall into the prostate and pulls back, bearing a small core of tissue. This is usually repeated six times to sample the entire region.

Men respond quite differently to a biopsy. "It brought me to tears," says sixty-six-year-old Bill. Seventy-nine-year-old Edgar, a retired career navy officer, represents the other end of the spectrum: "You feel a little pinch each time the doc shoots that thing. It's no big deal."

Most men sail through a biopsy without any lasting complications. A few, however, develop minor rectal bleeding that usually stops by itself. Some also develop a urinary-tract infection over the next few days, characterized by pain on urination and a fever. Antibiotics generally make short work of these infections. In addition, some men will see a spot or two of blood in semen or urine following the biopsy. This isn't a cause for alarm unless there's a lot of blood or it persists in the urine for several days. Semen may contain a bit of blood for up to a month.

In some centers, biopsies are performed perineally—through the patch of skin between the anus and scrotum. While this procedure requires no advance enemas or antibiotics, it does require a local anesthetic to numb the skin.

Pathology and Gleason Grading

Tissue samples taken during a biopsy are immediately dunked in preservative and stained with a special dye. Later they are sliced thinner than paper and examined under the microscope by a pathologist. He or she scans the biopsied tissue, looking for abnormalities. Normal, healthy prostate cells are round or oblong. They have smooth edges, are evenly spaced, and the nucleus takes up only a fraction of each cell's interior. Normal cells form glands that are packed together in a regular orientation. Cancer cells, by comparison, have irregular or jagged edges and the blue staining nucleus often fills the entire cell. "When you look at a slide and see lots of blue you immediately know the news won't be good," says Dr. Elizabeth Bailey, an MGH pathology fellow. Big, abundant nuclei mean the cells are dividing rapidly. The glands formed by these cells tend to invade and compress each other, looking jumbled rather than organized.

The pathologist uses this information to grade biopsied

tissue. The most commonly used system was devised by Dr. Lawrence Gleason, a pathologist and prostate-cancer researcher with the U.S. Veterans Administration. The system that bears his name provides extraordinarily important information on a tumor's potential for aggressive growth and metastasis.

In the Gleason scale, prostate biopsy samples are rated on a scale of 1 to 5 based on the gland's architecture. Samples that closely resemble normal prostate tissue earn a 1, those in which the glands are somewhat more spaced out earn a 2, those with a "cribriform" or sievelike pattern earn a 3, and tumors that no longer form glandlike tissue or that are an angry jumble of cells earn a 4 or 5, depending on how far from normal prostate tissue they appear. The pathologist assigns Gleason grades to the two most abundant types. These numbers are then added together, or reported with a plus sign. For example, a prostate biopsy that contains mostly normal-looking prostate tissue with a few spots of less-contained glands would receive a Gleason grade of 1 + 2, or 3/10.

Tumors with a Gleason grade of 2/10, 3/10, or 4/10 are called well differentiated. This means that the tumor looks similar to normal prostate tissue, and probably acts like it too. Well-differentiated tumors as a rule grow slowly, depend on testosterone for cell division, and stay confined to the prostate for a long time. Tumors graded 8/10 and higher are called poorly differentiated because they no longer resemble prostate tissue in looks or activity. They tend to grow quickly, spread aggressively to other parts of the body, and aren't as dependent on testosterone for growth or cell division. Tumors that earn Gleason grades of 5/10, 6/10, and 7/10 are called moderately differentiated and lie somewhere in between.

Bone Scan

When cancer cells escape from the prostate, they commonly spread to the bones, especially those in the pelvis and spine. If malignant cells work their way into the bone marrow, they begin growing new tumors made of prostate-like cells. A bone scan can detect small tumors growing in or on the spine, pelvis, rib cage, thigh, or other bones. This test is like a whole-body Xerox copy that omits the skin and internal organs and records only the bones. Men with low PSAs and normal alkaline phosphatase tests usually don't need a bone scan, since it adds little extra diagnostic information.

Bone scans don't require much preparation. You'll be given an intravenous injection of radioactive technetium-99 an hour or two before the scan. This compound acts like calcium inside the body and gets taken up by the bones. For the scan itself, you will lie on a movable table beneath a camera that responds to blips of energy from radioactive particles rather than to light. Beginning at your head, the camera will scan side to side as the table moves beneath it. Eventually, your whole body gets "read."

Bone scans work like reverse X rays. Instead of high-energy beams being shot through the body and exposing a sheet of film, high-energy particles emitted by the bones themselves expose the film. A computer assembles all the energy blips the camera records and creates a picture of your skeleton (fig. 6.3). Wherever bones take up extra technetium, a bright or "hot" spot appears. Hot spots signal areas of fast growth. These may be metastatic tumors. But a healed fracture or inflammation caused by arthritis, infection, or other diseases also appears as hot spots.

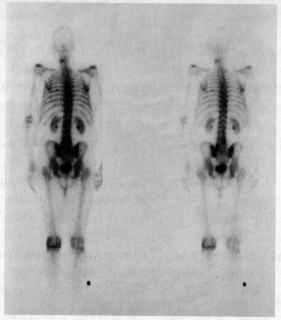

Figure 6.3. *A normal bone scan.*

Does the test make you radioactive? No. You will urinate away all the technetium that wasn't absorbed by the bones. And any that lingers in the bones or other tissues will quickly decay to a nonradioactive compound.

Computerized Tomography (CT) Scan

Only a minority of men really need a CT scan as part of the general workup for prostate cancer—those whose rectal exam or PSA suggests the tumor may be large and/or growing outside the prostate capsule; those with a poor or moderately differentiated tumor; or those who choose to have radiation therapy. For a variety of reasons, some urologists, medical centers, and HMOs include this test in their standard prostate-cancer evaluation, so don't immediately assume the worst when your physician suggests you have a scan.

These three-dimensional X rays serve several purposes: They can help determine whether or not a tumor has spread beyond the prostate into adjacent tissue or lymph nodes, and they provide an excellent picture of the kidney, liver, and nodes that can be quite helpful for a surgeon. The scan itself is much like having an X ray with a few minor differences. The first is that you'll probably have to drink some liquid the consistency of buttermilk that helps the stomach and intestines show up more clearly. Then you lie on a movable table that shuttles you through a cylindrical machine. As you pass through the middle, spinning generators shoot X-ray beams through your body at different angles. A computer records the images and creates a remarkably clear and lifelike picture (fig. 6.4).

Magnetic Resonance Imaging (MRI)

Another increasingly popular, though medically questionable, diagnostic tool for prostate cancer is the MRI (magnetic resonance imaging) scan. Like the CT scan, it, too, can sometimes detect metastatic cancer in lymph nodes or other tissues around the prostate. However, most studies show it adds little diagnostic or predictive information.

Instead of X rays or other radiation, an MRI sees inside the body with a magnetic field 10 million times more powerful than the earth's. So before entering the specially designed MRI room, leave your eyeglasses, watch, jewelry, and any other metal behind. As with a CT scan, a table

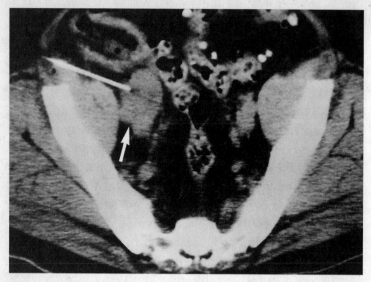

Figure 6.4. *The arrow on this CT scan points to a suspiciously enlarged lymph node. The white line going into the node is a needle used to take a tissue sample for biopsy.*

moves you into a doughnut-shaped machine. The magnetic field is turned on and off at regular intervals, accompanied by a loud bang that can get irritating. Other than that, you never feel a thing. The computer-generated picture that results clearly shows the internal organs and any suspicious areas.

Several researchers have been trying to improve MRI's accuracy by placing the magnetic field very close to the prostate using a magnetic generator inserted into the rectum, i.e., an endorectal coil. While the results are promising, even this adaptation is still far from accurate at detecting small tumors or those that have escaped the' gland.

Staging

All these tests have two basic goals. The rectal exam, PSA, and ultrasound-guided biopsy determine whether or not cancer is present. If so, information from the biopsy, bone scan, CT scan, PSA, and other tests attempt to *stage* the tumor. A cancer's stage is a function of three things: tumor size, location—confined to the prostate, extending to or through the capsule, or involving distant tissues—and Gleason grade. More than any other factor, staging points the way to the most appropriate treatment options and prognosis, which is a very general estimate of how you and your tumor will respond to treatment.

Physicians use two different but equivalent staging systems for prostate cancer. Some have adopted the Jewett-Whitmore scale which uses four basic categories, ranging from Stage A to Stage D. Others employ the international TNM (Tumor, Node, and Metastasis) scale. The table in figure 6.5 lists them side by side for comparison. When re-

Figure 6.5. Stages of prostate cancer

JEWETT-WHITMORE	TNM	
A-1	T-1a N0M0	Small focus of well or moderately differentiated cancer
A-2	T-1b N0M0	Cancer occurs in many areas or is poorly differentiated
B	T-2 N0M0	Palpable cancer confined to the prostate
C	T-3 N0M0	Cancer has spread through the capsule of the prostate or involves the seminal vesicles
D	T1, 2, or 3 N+M+	Metastatic cancer

ferring to a stage, this book gives the A to D stage with its counterpart in parentheses.

Stage A (T1) refers to all prostate cancers that are so small or so deep in the prostate that they can't be felt during a digital rectal exam. Stage A (T1) tumors are discovered either through examination of prostate "chips" removed during a transurethral resection of the prostate or because of an elevated PSA test. Stage B (T2) tumors are large enough to raise a bump on the gland but not so big they have spread beyond the capsule. Tumors in the stage C (T3) category are generally larger and have grown through the capsule into surrounding tissues. Stage D prostate cancer is metastatic cancer that has spread to one or more lymph nodes or to more distant sites such as bone. (In the TNM system, metastatic prostate cancer goes by several designations.)

The TNM system looks more complicated at first, but it really isn't. The marking T2cNOM1 in a medical chart is shorthand for a tumor that has spread throughout the entire prostate but has not perforated the capsule (T2c) with no tumor cells found in the lymph nodes (NO) and with a confirmed distant metastasis (M1).

Staging a tumor based on purely diagnostic tests is a bit like trying to figure out what's wrong with a car without ever opening the hood. You can start it up, listen to it idle, take it out for a spin around the block, and make some mighty good guesses. But each ping or chug or miss may have several possible causes that can't be pinned down until you look at the engine. Given the limited information that physicians get from diagnostic tests, they do a pretty good job of staging. Yet they often guess too low, a situation called understaging. After a prostatectomy—removal of the gland—when a surgeon has seen the prostate, its surrounding tissues, and lymph nodes, and a pathologist has examined samples under the microscope, as many as 25 percent of men find they have a more serious tumor than previously thought. This happens because a suspected stage B (T2) tumor was really poking through the capsule, making it a stage C (T3) tumor, or because one or more lymph nodes were found to contain tumor cells, or because tumor cells were found in the tissue surrounding the gland.

So keep in mind that when a physician says you have a stage A2 tumor, that's really a good working hypothesis. Chapter 7 describes how to use this information to pick the most appropriate treatment.

7

Making Your Decision

Physicians know how to handle most of the diseases that afflict us. Catch bacterial pneumonia and you'll take antibiotics and perhaps breathe oxygen through a mask. Develop insulin-dependent diabetes and the treatment invariably includes insulin shots and a strict diet. Unfortunately, there's no clearly defined, blue-ribbon, no-doubt-about-it treatment for prostate cancer. Researchers and clinicians just haven't figured out the best way to treat this increasingly common disease. Treatment options are hotly debated. Surgery can remove a tumor-bearing prostate. Radiation destroys cancer cells buried deep within the gland. Hormone therapy can slow the progress of the disease if it escapes the gland.

Any of these should, you would think, be more effective than doing nothing and letting the tumor grow unchecked. But even that's not necessarily true. Older men, especially those with a small, slow-growing, well-differentiated tumor confined to the prostate (stage A) who choose a no-treatment strategy called watchful waiting not only escape the side effects of treatment but appear to live just as long as those who opt for surgery or radiation.

What seems illogical on the surface stems from prostate-cancer cells' unique biological properties. As mentioned earlier, most of these tumors are the cancer world's slowpokes. Breast tumors double in size within six months or less; pancreatic tumors can grow even faster. A small, well-differentiated prostate tumor, by comparison, doubles every four years or longer. That means a tiny clump of cancer cells so small it can't be felt by a physician's finger will usually take five to ten years to develop into a tumor large enough to escape the prostate and spread to other parts of the body. Since the disease usually strikes men in their sixties and seventies, the ages at which men become more prone to death by heart attack, stroke, or other "natural causes," the majority of those afflicted with a small, well-differentiated tumor die *with* prostate cancer rather than *from* prostate cancer.

This slow growth may be the small silver lining in the dark cloud of prostate cancer. It could allow some older men, or those suffering from other serious illnesses, to essentially ignore prostate cancer and live out their lives without putting themselves through the pain, hassle, or potential complications associated with cancer treatment. Furthermore, it gives all men who have just been diagnosed with prostate cancer some time to get a second opinion, do some homework, and mull over their options. Taking one or two months to make a good decision won't likely threaten your health or your chances for getting rid of the cancer. More important, investing that time and effort will pay off in the long run by making you a more active partner in your treatment and recovery. "The time I spent talking with several physicians about my cancer and reading up on the disease made me understand why there weren't any easy answers," says Justin, a seventy-year-old dentist. "It also made me feel less helpless, like there was something that I could do for myself."

Treatment Strategies

Physicians currently recommend four basic treatment strategies for prostate cancer: surgery, radiation therapy, hormone therapy, and watchful waiting, sometimes called delayed therapy or expectant management. Chemotherapy, a key weapon in the fight against other cancers, isn't very effective against slow-growing tumors in the prostate. Each strategy has its defenders and critics; researchers continually debate the merits and drawbacks of all four. Unfortunately, scientifically valid, head-to-head comparisons haven't been done, making it impossible to tell which treatment is most effective in a particular situation.

The bottom line from hundreds of separate studies is this: For a small, well-differentiated stage A or stage B tumor completely confined to the prostate, surgery and radiation therapy appear to be equally effective at keeping men alive for five years. Beyond ten years, surgery offers a survival advantage over radiation therapy. For a select group of men, watchful waiting may equal surgery and radiation therapy over the short term, meaning under ten years. Beyond that time frame, however, the risk of metastatic disease steadily rises. For poorly differentiated tumors, which grow quickly and spread aggressively, watchful waiting isn't really an effective option. Finally, once a tumor metastasizes, hormone therapy emerges as the treatment of choice, though radiation and surgery or some combination of these three are often used.

This isn't the kind of decision you want to leave completely up to the experts. Your physicians undoubtedly have your best interests in mind, but you're the one who must live with the results and any treatment-related complications. A doctor's mission in life is curing people, and that usually involves aggressive therapy. But the best treatment for the cancer "may not be the best treatment for the patient," prostate-cancer pioneer Dr. Willet Whitmore once pointed out. This is especially true for early-stage prostate cancer—which causes no symptoms and doesn't interfere with daily life—because most men diagnosed with such a tumor are completely unaware they've been living with it. Treating this kind of tumor with radiation therapy or surgery, then, is like paying insurance. Even though you aren't suffering from any symptoms, you begin treatment in the hope that aggressive therapy now will prevent metastatic prostate cancer in the future. If today's cures were quick, painless, 100 percent effective, and didn't interfere with your life, then it would make perfect sense to pick one. But some men develop metastatic disease even after what appears to be successful surgery or radiation therapy. Both surgery and radiation require a substantial investment of time and energy, and both carry the risk of serious complications that can diminish the pleasure you get from life (fig. 7.1). In some cases, they can make your last years miserable. "Sometimes I wished that I still had the cancer instead of being incontinent from prostate surgery," says Henry, a seventy-six-year-old retired salesman, who changed his mind once he was fitted with an artificial sphincter that keeps him perfectly dry. To

Figure 7.1. Complications that may occur with radiation or surgery for cancer of the prostate

	RADIATION	SURGERY
Impotence	X	X
Incontinence	X	X
Diarrhea	X	
Frequent voiding	X	
Wound infection/drainage		X
Phlebitis		X
Rectal bleeding	X	
Incisional pain		X

complicate matters further, only a fraction of small prostate cancers ever grow large enough to threaten a man's health, meaning that radical treatment may sometimes be unnecessary for men seventy or seventy-five and older.

Perhaps some day researchers will devise an accurate test that tells the difference between a small tumor that will spread and one that won't. Until then, you're taking a calculated risk no matter what you choose. Pick watchful waiting and you gamble that you'll have several treatment-free, and thus side-effect-free, years before you die from a heart attack, stroke, or in your sleep. Choose surgery or radiation therapy and you gamble that the potential benefits—eradicating the cancer and adding extra months or years of life—outweigh the potential costs or the possibility of life-changing side effects.

Gathering Information

Making a good decision will take some work. You will have to consider your age, general health, and cancer stage. Then you need to factor in the survival rates for the four treatment options (surgery, radiation therapy, watchful waiting, and hormone-withdrawal therapy) and their potential for problematic complications or side effects. Finally, take a hard look at your own personal preferences and values about treatment and quality of life. "When there are no clear-cut treatment strategies, a man's values and preferences play an increasingly large role," says MGH internist Dr. Michael Barry, who has developed an interactive video to help men make decisions about prostate-cancer treatment. "People dealing with cancer sometimes put their preferences on the back burner and focus on getting rid of the disease. That's not necessarily the best approach for prostate cancer."

Some men want to do everything possible to eradicate a tumor. Others don't mind living with a small, slow-growing tumor that may never threaten their health because they fear treatment might interfere with their lifestyle. The risk of incontinence that accompanies surgery may steer a man toward radiation, even though surgery may have an edge when it comes to long-term survival. Or a man who hopes to have children or continue an active sex life might investigate treatments that won't interfere with his potency.

Thousands of men manage to make this choice every year. Some rely heavily on their urologists' recommendations. Others take a more active role and use that advice as one piece of the decision-making puzzle. Whatever method you use, it's important to feel confident about your choice before starting treatment. "My wife and I both felt good about the decision we made [to have a prostatectomy]," says Bob, a sixty-four-year-old engineer. "That kind of gave me a boost on some low days during my recuperation. Even today I don't look back with any regret, which is an important part of recovering from something like this."

Start by asking your physician questions. Don't hesitate to bring a written list of them to your appointments, and don't quit until you have the answers you need. After he or she lists your options and recommends a particular course of action, ask why: What are its advantages and disadvantages? What are other possible options? How do these others compare with the treatment he or she recommended? What published studies support that choice?

Next, do some homework. Reading this book is a good start. But the state of the art in medicine, and especially in prostate cancer, changes rapidly. New studies are published almost every month that may have an impact on the best way to treat this disease. And busy physicians don't always have time to read enough to stay completely up-to-date. The easiest way to tap into the latest thinking on prostate cancer (or any cancer, for that matter) is to pick up the phone and dial 1-800-4-CANCER. That's the number of the Cancer Information Service, a free service sponsored by the National Cancer Institute. The researchers you'll talk with aren't physicians, so they can't give you any advice or make recommendations. Instead, they are specialists at digging into the medical literature, mostly using a database called Physicians Data Query, or PDQ, which stores up-to-date information on cancer treatments. Tell the researcher as much as you can about your cancer. Be specific. Mention the tumor stage, Gleason grade, current PSA level, etc. He or she will then search through PDQ's database, print out information regarding your disease, and mail it to you within the week. PDQ also lists clinical trials under way around the country if you are seeking alternative treatment or your cancer is not responding to standard therapy.

You can search PDQ yourself, or the equally important MEDLINE, if you have electronic access to the National Library of Medicine's databases. Your public library may be able to link you up, and a number of hospitals, medical schools, and university libraries allow patients or members of the public to use their electronic access. MEDLINE lists and summarizes more than 47,000 medical articles published each month. Using key words like "prostate cancer," "radiation therapy," and "survival rate," a librarian can electronically dive into this ocean of information and, in a few minutes, surface with a printout listing recent articles on the topic you've asked about. Keep in mind that most of these will be hard to read, written by medical researchers for clinicians or other medical researchers. If you track down the articles themselves, read the abstract (a brief summary), the introduction, results, and discussion. These are usually the most helpful and readable sections.

Once you understand the key issues about treatment, seek out a second opinion. If the first physician you saw was a urologist, make an appointment with a radiation oncologist, a doctor who specializes in treating cancer with high-energy radiation. Or consult another urologist. He or she might not recommend the same options as the first one you saw. Don't be dismayed if two physicians recommend different treatments for your cancer. Not surprisingly, urologists—who are surgeons—tend to recommend surgery for an early-stage cancer while radiation oncologists tend to recommend radiation therapy. Another reason for disagreement could be that two physicians place different emphasis on individual factors such as your age or general health. To sort out conflicting medical opinions, talk to your internist or ask for a referral to a medical oncologist. These specialists are playing an increasingly important role in helping men clearly understand their options.

Men who have been treated for prostate cancer represent another excellent source of information. Many will share both good and bad experiences with you and give you a first-person account of what different treatments really involve. Most physicians just can't explain what it's like to recover from a prostatectomy, convey the personal embarrassment of total incontinence, or relate the psychological impact of impotence quite as graphically as those who have lived through them. If possible, try to talk with someone who has faced a similar-stage cancer as the one you are facing. Finding men to talk with isn't difficult. Your urologist, internist, or oncologist might be able to recommend several former patients. For a more independent source of referrals, call a local prostate cancer support group, such as Us-Too or Man-to-Man. (See the Resources section at the end of the book for addresses and telephone numbers.)

If you are computer savvy and have access to the Internet or to on-line services such as CompuServe, America Online, or Prodigy, try out the discussion groups multiplying in the ether. (See Resources for information on getting access to these groups.)

No matter how many others you've talked with, the ultimate decision must be yours. Physicians can tell you about statistical cure rates and the probability of side effects. Prostate-cancer survivors can describe their experiences. But what's right for others, or what national statistics show as the best treatment for a particular stage tumor, may not be right or best for you.

A final word of caution: Don't be seduced by rumors of surefire experimental therapies or articles reporting exciting new treatments. These new techniques are very tempting when compared with the modest and controversial successes of the tried-and-true therapies. But they rarely pan out in the long run. I tell my patients to investigate such therapies the same skeptical way they would an expensive, experimental car or a start-up company someone wanted them to invest in. Find out if the treatment has been tried before—many "new" treatments actually have long histories. If so, what were the results then? Why was it abandoned, and why is it making a comeback now? If it is a new treatment, ask how many men have used it, and how long have they been followed. Since prostate cancer can take up to ten or fifteen years to recur, two- or five-year survival rates mean very little.

Variables in Decision-Making

Here are the major variables you need to consider in making a decision about treatment.

Tumor Size

The size of a prostate tumor and whether or not it has spread beyond the gland determine, to a large extent, viable treatment options. As a general rule, small tumors completely contained inside the prostate can often be cured with aggressive local therapy (surgery or radiation) or they can be safely watched without treatment for a few years. Larger tumors that have spread beyond the gland usually aren't good candidates for surgery or radiation because it is impossible to find all the pockets of cancer cells and then destroy them.

Tumor size can sometimes be measured directly with ultrasound, or estimated using PSA levels. Researchers at Stanford University have shown that the higher the PSA, the larger the tumor. And a study from Washington University in St. Louis of 10,000 men age fifty and older related PSA level to tumor spread. The investigators found that 55 percent of the men with prostate cancer whose PSAs were above 10 had tumor cells extending beyond the prostate gland. If your PSA is much above this level, and your physician suggests "definitive" therapy such as a prostatectomy or radiation, make sure he or she clearly explains why. You don't want to go through either of these procedures only to have the cancer recur a few years later.

Tumor Differentiation

As I discussed earlier, not all prostate-cancer cells are created equal. Some form tumors that look almost exactly like normal, healthy prostate tissue. Others lose their "prostate-ness" and end up as an angry jumble of cell types and tissues. The difference is a crucial one. Tumors that resemble normal prostate tissue *act* like normal prostate tissue—they grow slowly, secrete normal fluids, and rarely migrate to other parts of the body. The others act like aggressive cancers, with rapid growth rates and a tendency to spread outside the gland.

It's up to the pathologist, an often unheralded member of the cancer-management team, to scrutinize cell samples taken during a biopsy or after a prostatectomy. He or she looks at thin slices of prostate or lymph-node tissue under a microscope, catalogs the predominant cellular architecture, and compares it with the way normal prostate tissue is supposed to look. The Gleason grading system (see Chapter 6) numerically tracks the resemblance, or lack of it. Tumors that retain the basic glandular structure of a healthy prostate earn a low Gleason score (4/10 or lower) and are called well differentiated. They grow slowly and don't aggressively leave the prostate. Poorly differentiated tumors (Gleason score of 8/10 or higher) tend to grow quickly and spread rapidly throughout the body. In a study of almost 3,000 men treated at Veterans Administration centers around the country, those with Gleason scores below 4/10 were far less likely to die from prostate cancer than those with Gleason scores greater than 8/10.

Tumor differentiation thus provides a key piece of information in deciding on prognosis and treatment, especially when it comes to localized tumors. A small, well-differentiated nodule could be a candidate for watchful waiting. A similarly sized but poorly differentiated tumor, by comparison, usually demands aggressive local therapy such as surgery or radiation since it is more likely to escape from the prostate.

Age

Age clearly influences treatment choices for prostate cancer in several important ways. One has to do with resilience—younger men tend to tolerate surgery or radiation therapy more readily than older men. Part of this, to be sure, is a function of health. Aging often brings with it a host of medical conditions such as diabetes, arthritis, poor circulation, or lung problems, all of which can slow down the whole system. There's no question that a fit, otherwise healthy seventy-year-old may tolerate surgery better than an overweight fifty-five-year-old smoker with high blood pressure. But when matched for health, older men heal more slowly and develop more treatment-related complications than younger men. Many urologists hesitate to do a prostatectomy on men seventy-five and older, and for good reason. A recent analysis of more than 10,000 men who had a radical prostatectomy showed that the risk of dying within thirty days of the procedure was very low for those under seventy-five, roughly one death per 500 operations. For men between seventy-five and seventy-nine, postoperative deaths rose to 1.4 per 100 operations. For men eighty and over, there were almost five deaths for every 100 operations. Since radiation therapy is much less traumatic than surgery, it may become the treatment of choice for older men.

There are exceptions to an "age rule." MGH urologist Dr. Alex Althausen recalls telling an otherwise healthy seventy-six-year-old man he was too old for a prostatectomy. "When he told me he was still taking care of both his parents, who were in their mid-nineties, I reconsidered. If family history meant anything, he still had at least another ten to fifteen years of life ahead of him." The man came through the operation with flying colors.

The real issue is much less straightforward: Is there an age beyond which a man with a small, well-differentiated tumor confined to the prostate (stage A or B) shouldn't put himself through the agony of treatment and potentially life-changing complications? Some men say no—the peace of mind that comes from removing or irradiating a tumor is worth the risk at any age. Others bet that they will live out their allotted years on earth before a tumor can harm them. As Dr. Willet Whitmore once put it: "Growing older is invariably fatal; prostate cancer is only sometimes so!"

New research from Europe and the United States supports the choice of watchful waiting for older men. In a 1994 study from the University of Chicago, for example, researchers followed men in their late sixties, seventies, and eighties who had been diagnosed with prostate cancer but who were not aggressively treated for the disease. Instead, they were regularly monitored with rectal exams and PSA tests. Men were offered hormone therapy only if the tumor began to spread. Ten years later, only 13 percent of those with stage A or B tumors had died as a result of their prostate cancer, while many more died from other causes. That's equivalent to survival rates following surgery or radiation therapy, and is roughly the same as a group of similarly aged men who did not have prostate cancer. In addition, watchful waiting caused no treatment-related impotence or incontinence, and didn't require daily visits to a radiation center or a several-week recovery period. The researchers concluded that watchful waiting was "a reasonable option for men with stage A or stage B clinically localized prostate cancer *if their life expectancy is ten years or less*" (emphasis added). They chose ten years as the cutoff point because beyond that more and more of the men began developing metastatic disease. Although this study should not be taken as the last word— several research teams have criticized this work—it clearly points out the important role life expectancy should play in your decision.

Predicting how many years you have left may seem morbid, even perverse. But such an exercise could provide an invaluable piece of information for picking the treatment that would serve you best. Census takers, statisticians, actuaries, and insurance adjusters routinely track survival rates and life expectancies. From their work have

Figure 7.2. Average number of years a man can expect to live

AGE	BLACK	WHITE
40	30.1	35.6
45	26.2	31.1
50	22.5	26.7
55	19.0	22.5
60	15.9	18.7
65	13.2	15.2
70	10.7	12.1
75	8.6	9.4
80	8.7	7.1
85+	5.0	5.2

SOURCE: U.S. Bureau of the Census. *Statistical Abstract of the United States,* 113th edition. Washington, D.C., Government Printing Office, 1993.

come tables like the one in figure 7.2, which shows the average number of years that men of different ages can expect to live. Keep in mind that these are averages compiled from hundreds of thousands of men. Like all averages, they can't predict anything for an individual, nor do they account for family history. If you are sixty-four and the men in your family live well into their nineties, take the estimate with a grain of salt. If, on the other hand, your male ancestors had fatal heart attacks before the age of sixty-five and at sixty-four you suffer from chronic high blood pressure, then living another decade may be a stretch. These statistics also don't take into consideration other health problems. Men with diabetes, or those who have had a heart attack or two have a lower life expectancy, on average, than otherwise healthy men.

If you have a small, well-differentiated, prostate-confined tumor and you realistically expect to live less than five years, watchful waiting may offer an attractive option, free from the side effects of surgery or radiation. If, on the other hand, you expect to live more than five to ten years, you have a large or poorly differentiated tumor, or your PSA is rising rapidly, then more aggressive therapy is in order.

Health

The healthier you are, the better a candidate you'll be for aggressive local treatment such as radiation therapy or surgery. Both carry some real risks, even for perfectly healthy men. Ailments such as heart disease or diabetes dramatically increase these risks. Obesity and smoking can also make treatment more hazardous. Perhaps even more to the point, poor health increases a man's chances of dying from something other than his prostate cancer.

Personal Preference

In addition to objective variables such as age, overall health, and cancer stage, don't ignore subjective ones like gut instinct or quality of life. Striking a balance between statistics and preferences should help you make a confident decision. Some of this confidence comes from knowledge. If you know beforehand that 50 percent of men who are potent before radiation therapy lose the ability to have an erection following treatment, and you choose that option, then temporary or permanent impotence shouldn't come as a surprise. So make sure you understand the downside of each treatment option. If your physician goes over them too quickly, ask again at your next appointment. Or ask a nurse, social worker, or member of a local prostate-cancer support group.

Knowing what's important to you and deciding what you want from treatment are also crucial. For some men, getting rid of every last cancer cell is of utmost importance. For others it's not being in pain. Some choose a particular treatment because it represents minimal hassle. "I chose surgery because I wouldn't drive into Boston five days a week for seven weeks for anything," says seventy-two-year-old John, a part-time chemical salesman, who opted against the radiation therapy regime. Sixty-one-year-old Harvey chose radiation therapy for a similar, personal reason: "I couldn't imagine being in the hospital for several days and recovering at home for another two to six weeks."

If you don't really have any strong preferences, go with what a doctor you trust suggests. If you do have strong preferences, make sure they become part of the initial plan—it's hard to work them in later, once treatment has already begun.

"Unless you feel good about your decision, you're always going to be second-guessing your doctor and thinking about what you could have done or should have done," says Bob, a fifty-five-year-old publishing company vice president who opted for a prostatectomy. "Then you never really get on with your life."

8

Surgery

There's something appealing to many men about the idea of surgery for prostate cancer. Removing a tumor along with the gland that contains it makes sense both logically and emotionally. A man doesn't need his prostate to live a long, healthy life, so losing it isn't anywhere near as troublesome as losing a kidney, a section of brain, or a lobe of lung tissue.

When cancer is confined to the prostate, surgically removing the gland often means the disease is gone for good. Time and time again researchers have compared the survival rate of a large group of men who chose a prostatectomy for gland-confined cancer with a similar-sized group of randomly selected men of the same age. Time and time again they have found virtually no difference in survival rates or death rates, evidence that surgery works. (Sometimes the researchers found that the men who underwent a prostatectomy actually lived longer! Don't get too excited, however. Surgery itself doesn't add years to life. As a group, candidates for surgery are generally healthier and have fewer other health problems than the average guy.)

If the operation, called a radical prostatectomy, was as simple and side-effect-free as removing a gallbladder, it would probably be *the* recommended treatment for this disease. Unfortunately, the prostate is tucked away deep in the pelvis. It completely surrounds the urethra, a tube vital for urination and reproduction. Nerves and blood vessels that control erections course over its surface. The operation is fairly long and can be bloody. It requires a four-day hospital stay, and full recovery can take six weeks. The procedure causes impotence in somewhere between 30 and 70 percent of the men who opt for it, depending on whose statistics you read. Virtually every man is incontinent for a short time after the surgery. National statistics suggest that total incontinence, the complete inability to control urination, persists in 5 to 10 percent of men, while partial incontinence may plague a quarter or more.

Choosing Radical Prostatectomy

Despite these risks, more and more men are choosing a radical prostatectomy to fight stage A and B prostate cancer. In 1970, only 10 percent of men with a localized tumor underwent a radical prostatectomy. Today, according to a Gallup poll sponsored by the American Foundation for Urologic Disease, more than 50 percent choose this treatment option. Here are some of their reasons:

• "As a physician, I couldn't live knowing that I had a tumor growing inside me," says Justin, a seventy-year-old dentist.

• "If you have radiation and the cancer comes back, you can't get radiation again. But if you have surgery and it returns, then radiation is still an option. I liked knowing there was a fallback," says Bernard, a sixty-four-year-old investment counselor.

• "It just seemed like the best way. I wanted to get rid of the cancer, have it removed. I figured I'd worry about incontinence and erection kits later," says Bob, a fifty-five-year-old publishing vice president.

The operation itself has evolved in the last decade. Until the late 1970s, prostatectomy was performed through an incision between the scrotum and anus, what surgeons call the perineal route. That approach made it tough to see the prostate and surrounding tissue, especially lymph nodes and nerves. Any man who could have an erection following that operation was a medical surprise.

In the late 1970s, Johns Hopkins urologist Dr. Patrick Walsh and his colleagues revolutionized the field of prostate surgery. They improved the retropubic technique, which starts with an incision made from belly button to pubic bone. This approach makes it easier to identify crucial blood vessels and control bleeding, so surgeons can see exactly what they are doing. At the same time, Walsh and Dutch anatomist Dr. Pieter Donker made a startling anatomical discovery: Nerves and blood vessels responsible for controlling erections (the neurovascular bundles) don't enter the prostate, as urologists had believed for decades, but run along either side of the gland's capsule, using it for support on their way to the penis.

Thus was born what Walsh calls the "anatomical approach to radical prostatectomy" and what the media and most men call the nerve-sparing radical prostatectomy. Using the retropubic approach, a surgeon can carefully trace the neurovascular bundle, gently tease it away from the prostate capsule, and leave it intact while removing the gland. Since 1984, when news of the nerve-sparing approach began spreading among surgeons and through the popular media, the number of prostatectomies performed each year has increased 600 percent. Preliminary ten-year survival data from the first group of men to have a nerve-sparing prostatectomy show the procedure to be as effective at controlling prostate cancer as the perineal approach.

Keep in mind that the nerve-sparing approach doesn't *guarantee* postprostatectomy erections. The goal of surgery is to remove the visible tumor plus a zone of healthy tissue around the gland to capture any cancer cells that may have escaped from the tumor. If the tumor is small and contained well inside the prostate's tough outer covering, then simply removing the gland should suffice. But if the tumor comes close to the capsule, or has begun growing into or through it, the surgeon must remove a wider margin of tissue. This often includes the nerves and blood vessels that make erections possible. Sometimes the surgeon can preserve both neurovascular bundles, sometimes just one, and sometimes neither.

If you are considering a nerve-sparing prostatectomy, discuss this point with your surgeon. Make sure you clearly understand that this technique offers the possibility, not the certainty, of potency following the operation. You also need to know that erections after surgery may be softer or less long-lasting than they were before surgery. In a 1994 report to the American College of Surgeons, prostate cancer expert Dr. William Catalona from Washington University in St. Louis said that most men lose some erectile stiffness following a radical prostatectomy. "Only the youngest, healthiest men have perfectly normal erections after surgery," he said. In an earlier study, he assessed the return of sexual function in 295 men who were potent before surgery and whose tumors allowed for preserving one or both neurovascular bundles. Overall, 63 percent of those who had the bilateral nerve-sparing procedure regained erections, and only 41 percent of those with the unilateral procedure. Older men and those with more-advanced tumors did worse, younger men and those with less-advanced tumors did better, reported Dr. Catalona.

To ensure the best results you can possibly get, put yourself in the hands of a board-certified urologist. (See Resources.) They are physicians who have satisfied demanding requirements set by the American Board of Urology and have qualified as specialists in treating diseases of the male and female urinary system and the male reproductive system. The success of any operation depends in large part on a surgeon's skill. This is especially true for a tricky one like the nerve-sparing prostatectomy. As with any skill from fly-fishing to welding, experience and opportunity are the best teachers. Ask a potential surgeon how many of these operations he or she has done before, or how many he or she does a month. As a rough guide, look for someone who has performed more than seventy-five or 100 nerve-sparing prostatectomies and does several each month.

Your best bet is to find a surgeon at a large center where this kind of procedure must be done over and over. Here's why: Some recent data from around the country suggest that total incontinence and impotence rates following radical prostatectomy are 5 to 10 percent and above 70 percent, respectively. But in our department at MGH, less than one-half of 1 percent of men are totally incontinent following a radical prostatectomy, about 3 percent have significant stress incontinence when straining with a full bladder, and 15 percent occasionally lose a few drops when they cough or sneeze. Only about 8 men per 100 are wearing pads one year after surgery. The same trend applies to potency. Sixty percent of our patients have some erectile function, but only 30 to 40 percent can have sexual intercourse without some sort of aid.

When looking for a surgeon, don't let anyone hurry you into the operation. Since prostate cancer usually grows slowly, it's the rare man who requires an immediate prostatectomy. Before agreeing to the procedure, make sure you are comfortable with the idea of having your prostate removed. It can't be put back, and the side effects can't always be corrected. I can't emphasize enough how important it is to ask questions, read up on the subject, and then ask more questions. A potential surgeon who doesn't take the time to talk with you, talks down to you, or tries to rush you through this stage of your investigation may lack the compassion and understanding you'll want after surgery. Take the time to get a second opinion if you feel you need one. On the other hand, don't dawdle for weeks and weeks, especially if your tumor is moderately or poorly differentiated. "I never got the sense there was any urgency about beginning treatment," says Bruce, a fifty-eight-year-old minister. "So I thought things over, procrastinated a bit and waited until the time seemed right to go ahead with treatment—about five months after I got the diagnosis. But by then the tumor had broken through the outside of the gland and I had to go have radiation therapy after surgery."

For treating early-stage cancer confined to the prostate, surgery makes good sense for a number of reasons:

• Taking out the entire gland has the potential of completely removing the tumor, assuming that no cells have migrated to other tissues or organs. Fully 90 percent of men with stage A1 (T1a) or stage B1 (T2a) tumors who choose a radical prostatectomy die years later of something other than their prostate cancer. Or put another way, cancer recurs in 10 percent of men with early-stage tumors following a prostatectomy. For stage A2 (T1b) or stage B2 (T2b), approximately 75 percent live ten years or more.

• Surgery offers a psychological advantage that neither radiotherapy nor watchful waiting can offer—the sense that the cancer has been taken out of the body.

• During and after a prostatectomy, a surgeon and pathologist actually see the prostate and can examine it to determine how extensive the tumor is. Lymph nodes removed during the operation can also be examined to see if the disease has spread beyond the gland. With radiation therapy and watchful waiting, a special procedure called laparoscopic lymphadenectomy can be performed to get a similar look at the lymph nodes. But this is rarely done.

• If some tumor cells remain in the body following surgery, radiation therapy can follow within a few weeks. (The reverse, surgery following radiation therapy, is not recommended since it requires an extraordinarily skillful and experienced surgeon and carries with it a very high complication rate. See page 163.) Hormone therapy can also be started following surgery if the potential for metastatic spread is there.

Like all treatments, a radical prostatectomy has its drawbacks:

• It significantly disrupts your life. Most men stay in the hospital for four days following a prostatectomy, then recuperate at home for another three to six weeks. Some men find it difficult to give up that large a chunk of time, and opt for radiation therapy instead.

• A prostatectomy is a major, major operation that stresses some men so much they die from a heart attack or stroke. On average, this happens in less than one operation per 100. Young, otherwise healthy men having their operation at the Massachusetts General Hospital or other large medical center, with an experienced surgeon, face an even lower risk—closer to one per 10,000 operations. For men seventy-five and older, many of whom have heart and other health problems, as many as eight of 100 die within three months of a prostatectomy. (Here again, these numbers are national averages. At large medical centers death following a prostatectomy happens far less often.) Other postoperative complications include infection, blood clots getting stuck in the lungs, and damage to the rectum.

• Some potentially life-changing side effects accompany the operation. As mentioned above, incontinence and/or impotence affect many men who choose to have a prostatectomy. For some, these conditions gradually disappear; for others they last for life. Potency aside, *all* men permanently lose the ability to father a child after prostatectomy. Other potential side effects include the formation of impassable kinks in the urethra called strictures.

Preparing for Surgery

One to Four Weeks Before

Just as you'd spend time planning a vacation, you'll need to prepare for a prostatectomy.

In the hospital, physicians, nurses, and other staffers will take care of your every need. After the operation, all you'll have to do is focus on healing, walking, and learning to live with a catheter coming out of your penis. Back at home, though, things aren't necessarily so simple. You need to eat, get from place to place, take care of your catheter, and start getting back to normal. If you have a partner and you're retired, then you have help and plenty of time to recover. But if you are widowed, divorced, single, or otherwise living alone, you'll need to arrange for someone—children, relatives, friends, a visiting nurse—to help out for several weeks. If you're employed, you will need to arrange several weeks of medical leave and perhaps a temporarily modified job when you return, one without heavy lifting or straining.

For at least a short time following surgery, you probably won't have much control over your bladder. Incontinence can be irritating, embarrassing, messy, and emotionally devastating. An organization called Help for Incontinent People (HIP) offers information on dealing with incontinence, everything from simple exercises meant to build up the pelvic muscles to advice on what kind of pads or adult diapers to use. Since it takes several weeks to get this information, call HIP at 800-BLADDER as far in advance of surgery as possible.

You may want to store some of your own blood to replace what's lost during surgery. This process, called autologous blood donation, takes two or three hour-long visits to the hospital or local blood bank. The visits are usually spaced a week apart, and a pint of blood is collected each time. Most men who do this are given a prescription for iron pills to ensure that new red blood cells are made quickly and efficiently. Iron pills tend to darken the stool, so don't be alarmed by blackish feces. They can also cause mild constipation, which can be overcome by drinking plenty of fluids, eating high-fiber foods, and taking a stool-softening laxative.

After a prostatectomy, you won't be able to father a child by normal sexual intercourse *even if your erections return*. Prostate removal is the ultimate vasectomy. In addition to eliminating secretions thought to be necessary for fertilization, it also causes dry ejaculations. If you hope to have a child after a prostatectomy, you'll have to rely on the wonders of modern infertility medicine. Sperm banking is one way to preserve the option of future fatherhood. Semen frozen to −196 degrees Celsius can be thawed out months or years later and used in artificial-insemination techniques like in vitro fertilization. For information on this, look in the Yellow Pages under "sperm bank" for a facility in your area. If none are listed, you can get information from Resolve, a national organization that helps those with fertility problems (see Resources).

Many hospitals preadmit men bound for a prostatectomy. This means going through a battery of tests one or two weeks before surgery—blood studies, chest X ray, an electrocardiogram to check the heart, a visit with an anesthesiologist or nurse anesthetist. If possible, you should meet with the nurses who will take care of you during your in-hospital recuperation and take a tour of the floor. Meeting beforehand with a respiratory therapist to learn deep-breathing exercises used after the operation would also be most helpful.

The final ten days before surgery, make sure you don't take aspirin for aches or pains. This common home remedy prevents blood from clotting as quickly as it should, and it could lead to excess bleeding during and after the prostatectomy. If you regularly take aspirin, make sure your surgeon knows this in advance. He or she may switch you to something less likely to interfere with clotting. Nonsteroidal anti-inflammatory medications such as motrin or ibuprofen don't have the same anticlotting effect as aspirin and can be taken up until the day of surgery.

The Night Before

The final countdown to surgery begins with dinner, your last meal before the operation. No food or drink is allowed for ten hours before surgery because an empty stomach decreases the possibility of anesthesia-induced vomiting. Your surgeon will probably give you some antibiotics to reduce the potential for postoperative infection. Sometime before bed, you will need to drink several glasses of a special bowel-cleansing fluid or take a laxative and give yourself an enema. By clearing the intestines and rectum of digested food or feces, these measures reduce the chance of bacteria spilling into the abdominal cavity in case the rectum or intestines are nicked or torn during the operation.

The Big Day

Most hospitals and medical centers ask you to check in very early on the morning of surgery. Bring to the hospital whatever you think will make the stay more comfortable. If you have favorite pajamas, slippers, or robe, pack them along. They're bound to make you feel more comfortable when walking around than the standard-issue johnnies. (Other suggestions are usually listed in the preadmission materials most hospitals give their surgery patients.) Some men bring a fat book or two, others enjoy the leisure of watching daytime television, still others bring along some work. "We've had men come in with portable computers and fax machines, and set up temporary offices in their hospital rooms," says urology nurse Mary McDonough.

You will meet several doctors, nurses, and others responsible for your care. Each one may ask you the same set of questions. Irritating though this may be, answer patiently—they all need this information, and it reduces the potential for miscommunication if you tell each person the facts. Once you've been admitted and prepped for surgery, a nurse or orderly will wheel you down to the operating room. Once in the brightly lit operating theater, be prepared for what may seem like noisy confusion. It's not, just the bustle of teams preparing themselves and you for the next few hours. Here are the key players and what they do:

• The surgeon does the operating. He or she might be assisted by another surgeon or a surgical resident, an M.D. who is completing special training in surgery.

• The scrub nurse keeps track of all instruments and equipment used during the procedure—a critical job!

• The circulating nurse helps get you ready for surgery once you're in the operating room.

• The anesthesiologist (and perhaps an anesthesiology resident) administers the drugs that keep you unconscious and unaware during the operation. He or she also monitors your heartbeat, blood pressure, the amount of oxygen dissolved in the bloodstream, and other vital signs.

Once you and the operating-room team is ready, the anesthesiologist will drip a powerful sedative through the

IV line. A deep, unconscious sleep comes before you can count to ten. Once you are out, the anesthesiologist slides a breathing tube down your relaxed throat and into the top of your lungs. It delivers a mixture of oxygen and anesthetic gas and removes carbon dioxide and other waste gases. Almost simultaneously you'll be washed from chest to testicles with antibacterial soap, shaved, and "painted" with a strong antiseptic solution. Again, all these measures aim to reduce the potential for infection during and after surgery. Finally, a Foley catheter, which is illustrated in Chapter 3 (figs. 3.5 and 3.6), will be inserted through the tip of your penis and into the urethra.

The actual operation begins with the surgeon making an incision from belly button to pubis, the bone at the base of the penis. Metal retractors hold the layers of muscle and fat aside, creating an opening through which to work. The first order of business is removing the lymph nodes that trap and filter fluids seeping around the prostate. If cancer cells escape from the gland, these are a common stopping place. Once removed, the lymph nodes are preserved and sent to the pathology department for a thorough examination.

With the prostate in view, the surgeon next secures blood vessels that supply the prostate. This can be done with suture material and scissors or a special instrument called an electrocautery scalpel. It uses heat to slice through tissue, while at the same time sealing off small veins and arteries. Isolating the prostate's blood supply is a crucial step that determines whether or not a transfusion will be needed.

Once the prostate has been disconnected from its blood supply, the seminal vesicles are teased away from the rectum. Then the surgeon cuts through the tough connective tissue that anchors the prostate and keeps it from bouncing around when you run or jump. This basically frees the gland from everything but the urethra and base of the bladder. Just as it is impossible to slide an apple off its core, so it's impossible to slide the prostate off the urethra. The surgeon must slice through the urethra above and below the prostate. These two cuts sever the gland's link to the body, and it can be lifted out and deposited in a dish of preservative and sent to the pathologist.

Next the urethra must be lined up with the bladder so the tube runs straight, without twists or kinks. The matching ends are then sewn together using the catheter as support to form a watertight seal, or anastomosis in surgeon lingo. With this step, the operation winds down. The surgeon places a drainage tube in the pelvis that will collect blood, lymph, or other fluids that may gather in the prostatic space. It emerges from one side of the abdomen below the belly button. Finally, he or she sews up the incision or closes it with surgical staples.

About this time, the anesthesiologist shuts off the flow of anesthetic gas and you begin floating back to consciousness. Once you're definitely awake and breathing on your own, he or she will remove the breathing tube and unhook you from the monitors. Then it's on to the recovery room, where one or more nurses will make sure your breathing, pulse, and vital signs return to normal. They also keep an eye on how much urine collects in the Foley bag and how much blood comes out of the drainage tube. You'll drift in and out of sleep and might not remember anything until you're back in your hospital room.

Recovery

Day one is generally lost in the drowse of narcotic-assisted sleep. Nurses, doctors, and visitors fade in and out as you do. Tubes take care of most of your needs—an IV line supplies nutrients and fluids, the catheter drains away urine, the drainage tube draws away blood and lymph from where your prostate used to be. The intravenous line may be connected to a device called the PCA (patient-controlled analgesia) pump. It lets you give yourself a dose of pain medication whenever you need it, rather than waiting for a scheduled dose or whenever you can get a nurse's attention. The key to dealing with pain is nipping it in the bud rather than letting it build up and then fighting it. So if you are in pain, *push the button*. There's no need to worry about addiction since a "lockout" feature automatically prevents overdosing. After two or three days of either the pump or injections, you'll be switched over to oral pain medications. The same thing applies here. Don't be macho and tough out pain; doing so hurts only yourself.

After surgery, your body produces an excess of blood-clotting factors. That's good, because it helps stop bleeding in the area where your prostate once resided. But it has a downside. Small clots can form more easily, especially in inactive legs. If clots break away and begin circulating, they can damage the lungs or cause a stroke. Long before you think you're ready to get up, a nurse or physician will encourage, even insist, that you take a few steps around the room. Walking is great insurance against blood clots, because as leg muscles work they squeeze the veins and keep blood circulating. If you absolutely can't move, you may find a doctor or nurse rolling onto your legs a pair of pulsating stockings that mechanically squeeze blood back toward the heart.

At first you won't believe you can walk around with an intravenous line attached to your arm and a Foley catheter coming out of your penis. But with the IV and Foley bags hooked to a pole on wheels, you'll soon get the hang of it. The Foley *won't slip out*, even though it always feels ready to do so. "You could tell the guys who were just beginning their recovery because they walked the hospital hall so carefully and slowly," says John, a seventy-two-year-old part-time salesman. "But after a few tries, you learn how to hold yourself and realize that thing is attached pretty good, and you can kind of forget it."

The deep breathing exercises you learned before surgery come in handy during recovery. Most men take shallow breaths after a prostatectomy for the simple reason that each one hurts. Shallow breathing allows small air sacs in the lungs to collapse. This condition, known as atelectasis, sets the stage for pneumonia. The exercises can save you from spending extra time in the hospital fighting pneumonia or some other lung infection. Taking deep, regularly spaced breaths also stretches tight abdominal muscles and can gradually reduce the pain of breathing.

Eating may not be high on your list of priorities immediately after surgery, but it's best to try. Start with liquids and then work your way up to mashed potatoes or Jell-O, then to chicken or stew. But in order to keep food down, your bowels have to be working. That can take a few days, especially if you are taking narcotics for pain. (A switch of pain medication can sometimes bring an end to constipation.) Not too long ago, most hospitals required a bowel movement before letting you leave. "I was having trouble with that," says Justin. "I really wanted to go home, but just couldn't have that bowel movement. When it finally came, it was as satisfying as the most intense orgasm I ever had." While that's no longer a requirement, some men feel more comfortable having that first bowel movement in the hospital.

The biggest changes come during the first three or four days of recovery. You'll go from feeling like something the cat dragged in to a shade of your old self. Each succeeding day you'll probably feel better and better.

Recovery at Home

You leave the hospital a different man from the one who entered: prostateless, wearing a stripe of adhesive strips, stitches, or staples on your shaved abdomen, constantly adjusting a tube coming out your penis, perhaps a few pounds lighter, and minus a spring in your step. Returning home may be a blessed relief—you'll sleep in your own bed, eat at your own table, maybe putter around your backyard. You won't, however, pee in your own pot, at least not for another two to three weeks. That's how long the Foley catheter stays in, to give the resealed urethra time to heal.

The biggest challenge for men following a prostatectomy is living with the Foley. It's uncomfortable, protrudes from the penis, leaks now and then, and must be attached to a collection bag (see Chapter 3, fig. 3.6). It requires constant attention and must be kept scrupulously clean. Make sure you follow diligently the instructions your doctor or nurse gave you about caring for the Foley. A little inattention can earn you a nasty, hard-to-shake bladder or urinary-tract infection.

You'll leave the hospital with two collection bags. A

larger one for at-home or nighttime use can be hooked to a chair, bed rail, or night stand. A smaller "leg bag" can be worn strapped to the leg and fits invisibly under most loose pants. (See figure 3.6 on page 51) Keeping that leg bag in place, however, can be a real challenge. With a bit of tinkering, you can devise your own system. Or call a local prostate-cancer support group. The men there have all worn Foleys and can pass on some useful tips.

Everything should go smoothly at home if you keep telling yourself you've just been through major surgery. Take it easy. Don't try to get back to your presurgery weight or level of activity right away. A safe, smooth recovery takes a big pinch of common sense and attention to a few details:

- Walk often, but start with short distances. A circuit of your downstairs every hour might make a good start. Increase the distance you walk each day. Avoid repeated stair climbing when possible for the first four to six weeks. If you are used to more vigorous daily exercise, check with your physician to plan what you can and can't do. Avoid motions or activities that put pressure on the abdomen—sit-ups, lifting heavy objects, swinging a golf club.
- Shower all you want, but refrain from full immersion baths until after the catheter has been removed.
- Do a few Kegel exercises (see Chapter 13, page 259) whenever possible. The stronger you make your external sphincter muscle, the more bladder control you will have when the catheter is removed.
- Don't drive, especially not until you are Foley-free. The catheter can interfere with your reaction times and movements.
- Avoid long car or plane trips, or any activity that

keeps you sitting in one position for long periods of time. Such immobility can put undue pressure on the urethra and cramp your circulation. Try to move around as often as possible.

Your body will let you know it can handle more activity or tell you when you've done too much. Above all, don't ignore pain and tough it out. Pain is usually a warning signal that something is wrong. Pay attention to it. For the persistent pain of surgical recovery don't be afraid to take the drugs your doctor has prescribed. If you feel sharp, constant leg pain, or constant pain in and around the incision, or feel feverish, give your doctor or nurse a call. These may be warning signs of an infection or other problem that needs prompt attention.

Don't be alarmed if the urine in your Foley bag has a pinkish tinge, or a small blood clot appears there now and then. A little bit of bleeding is entirely normal. If, however, the pinkish color fails to disappear after a few days or deepens with time rather than fades, call your doctor or nurse. And if the Foley ever falls out, a rare occurrence, don't try to replace it. Put on a urine-absorbing pad, call your doctor or nurse, and have an expert reinsert it if necessary.

Approximately ten days after the operation, your surgeon should be calling with news you've been waiting for—the pathologist's report. "You had clear margins" or "Your cancer was confined to the prostate" means that the tumor did not penetrate the capsule, no cancer cells were found in the area of tissue surrounding the gland, nor did any appear in the removed lymph nodes. While this does not guarantee that the surgeon removed every last cancer cell from your body, it certainly improves the odds of remaining cancer-free for the rest of your life.

Despite the best staging tests known, surgery and the pathology tests that follow sometime reveal that cancer has spread beyond the gland. Roughly 25 percent of men who thought they had stage A (T1) or stage B (T2) cancer before surgery learn afterward they have stage C (T3) or stage D cancer. The former means the tumor penetrated the capsule or cancer cells appeared in tissue surrounding the prostate. If the tumor's spread appears confined to the area directly around the prostate, both radiation and hormone therapy may be appropriate choices. If, however, lymph nodes test positive for cancer—stage D—then hormone therapy may be a better choice. Some urologists prefer to "watch and wait" at this point until it is clear that there are also other metastases elsewhere.

Postprostatectomy radiation therapy may or may not be recommended if the margins are positive. If it is, it begins one to two months after surgery. It takes approximately thirty-five treatments spread out over seven weeks, much the same as for primary radiation (see Chapter 9). Hormone therapy can begin right away or be deferred for a while. Some physicians recommend starting before symptoms appear in an effort to delay them. Others recommend waiting as long as possible to avoid the complications of hormone therapy, primarily impotence and a waning interest in sex (see Chapter 12).

Two to three weeks after surgery, another red-letter day arrives—Foley-removal day. "At the time, I thought that was one of the best days of my life," says Mike, a seventy-three-year-old former draftsman. Once the balloon holding the catheter snugly inside the bladder is deflated, the catheter slides right out with only a slight burning sensation. After that, you're free from the annoying plastic tube and ready to begin urinating on your own. Make sure you bring adult diapers or absorbent pads to this appointment. You might not have any control over your bladder, and urine will dribble out of your penis despite your best mental and physical efforts to stop it. If it happens, get used to it; it will be a fact of life for a few weeks if you're lucky, for much longer if you aren't. If you haven't been practicing Kegel exercises (see page 259) beforehand, this is a real incentive to start.

Assuming you are continent and potent, and the tumor was confined to the gland, this visit closes the crisis phase of your prostate-cancer experience. Put it behind you and get on with the rest of your life. But make sure that your plans for the next fifteen years include follow-up visits. Prostate cancer can, and does, recur even after a small stage A or stage B tumor was successfully removed. About one in ten men face this grim aftershock. A periodic PSA and rectal exam are really all that are needed. Following a prostatectomy, below-normal PSAs suggest no recurrence, while a rising PSA sounds an early warning.

Complications of Surgery

Every operation has its unintended consequences, things that didn't exactly go according to the script—an infected incision after a hernia repair, irritating tightness around the mouth after a facelift, stiffness in the knee following arthroscopy. Several kinds of complications accompany radical prostatectomies. Some are specific for prostatectomy, others can occur with any kind of surgery. Some appear right away, others develop over time. While complications hit even the most healthy men who have surgery, they are more likely to develop in older men or men with heart disease, diabetes, or high blood pressure. Smokers and overweight men also experience more than their share of complications.

General, Surgery-Related Complications

INFECTION

While we tend to think of hospitals as sterile, antiseptic places, the very fact that they admit patients with serious infections actually makes them havens for microbes. A recent study suggests that one out of six people who are hospitalized end up with a hospital-transmitted infection. Despite the best efforts of your surgeon and nurses, bacteria and other germs can sneak into the open abdomen or incision and set up an infection. In most cases, this means a fever, modest discomfort, a course of antibiotics, and perhaps an extra day or two in the hospital. On occasion, though, the bugs that cause hospital infections resist standard antibiotics and can trigger a life-threatening illness.

PNEUMONIA

A number of men develop pneumonia following a prostatectomy. This infection often appears when the lungs are somehow weakened. Anesthetic gases can compromise the lungs by dissolving in the lining and causing small air sacs to stick together. Shallow breathing—a common response to chest and abdominal pain after surgery—further intensifies the problem. Collapsed air sacs provide a refuge for bacteria to grow and multiply. Those deep-breathing exercises that nurses nag their postprostatectomy patients to do can help prevent pneumonia. Once it appears, antibiotics can usually fight off the infection. In severe cases, oxygen therapy may also be needed.

EMBOLISM

The body's response to the stress of surgery and the inevitable lying around that follows an operation combine to promote the formation of blood clots, especially in the pelvis and legs. When one of these breaks away and blocks an artery in the lungs, it is called a pulmonary embolism. Breathing becomes difficult and death can sometimes follow. Clots that block blood vessels in the brain can cause a stroke. Exercise, it turns out, is one of the best ways to prevent blood clots. That's why your nurses and doctors will strongly encourage you, or even hound you, to begin walking around your room or the hospital corridors as soon as possible. Contracting muscles squeeze veins and arteries and keep blood moving through them. If you won't be able to walk for a few days, your nurse may dress your legs in a pair of elastic socks that pulse on their own, gently massaging the legs and minimizing the chance of a clot.

DIARRHEA, CONSTIPATION, OR OTHER GI DISCOMFORT

In order to see the prostate, a surgeon must move the intestines out of the way, then replace them before sewing up the incision. This pushing and shoving can disrupt intestinal function. Pain medication and anesthetic agents can also alter bowel function and cause constipation. Antibiotics can do just the opposite and cause diarrhea. Rest, healing, proper diet, and drugs all help quell gastrointestinal discomfort. Diarrhea and colon inflammation persist, however, in a small percentage of men following prostatectomy due to an overgrowth of bacteria. Special antibiotics are the only way to eradicate them.

Prostatectomy-Related Complications

INCONTINENCE

Every man suffers some inability to hold his water following a prostatectomy. For most, this is a temporary condition that gradually resolves itself as nerves and muscles return to their presurgery shape. This return of urinary continence can take as long as two years. Somewhere between 0.5 and 10 percent of men are completely incontinent after a radical prostatectomy, and 15 to 50 percent suffer from stress incontinence—leaking small squirts of urine upon coughing, sneezing, sitting, lifting heavy objects, or other activities that suddenly compress the bladder. Why are the ranges so wide? The low numbers come from the best-known and most widely respected prostate-cancer centers in the country. The higher numbers come from a survey of Medicare records and probably reflect results at hospitals where few prostatectomies are performed each year. Both are true, meaning it is impossible to predict exactly what your risk for incontinence is. It depends on your health, presurgery urinary control, and the skill of your surgeon.

Normally, two circular muscles called sphincters control urine flow. One surrounds the urethra as it leaves the bladder, the other encircles it near the anus, just before it enters the penis. In addition, the prostate puts a constant pressure on the urethra, squeezing and compressing it, providing further resistance against urine flow. When your bladder is full, or when you decide to urinate before taking a long drive, a signal from the brain relaxes the sphincters and the pressure in the bladder overcomes any prostate-generated resistance. A prostatectomy usually removes two of those controls, leaving just the lower sphincter. Immediately after surgery it isn't strong enough to take on the entire task of controlling urine flow. With time and exercise, many men build up this muscle and learn simple tricks to avoid incontinence. In others the muscle was damaged or removed during surgery in order to dig out all of the tumor, leaving little musculature for urine control.

Through interviews and questionnaires, Dr. Mark Litwin has gathered data on life after prostatectomy from hundreds of men. He finds that men are far more troubled by urinary incontinence after a prostatectomy than they are by sexual impotence. "Impotence is a private thing that many men learn to deal with," said Dr. Litwin, assistant professor of urology and public health at UCLA's Jonsson Comprehensive Cancer Center. "But incontinence can be very public—even a little leakage can be embarrassing. And it's humiliating to be an adult in diapers."

Chapter 13 discusses the impact of incontinence as well as temporary and permanent solutions for controlling it.

IMPOTENCE

As described earlier, a nerve-sparing prostatectomy can sometimes preserve a man's ability to have an erection. In a hospital like Massachusetts General, where surgeons routinely perform this procedure, around 60 percent of men who are potent before surgery and whose tumors don't come close to the neurovascular bundles can expect their erections to return after surgery. (Though perhaps the erections won't be as firm or as long-lasting as they had been prior to surgery—only half or so of men who keep some erectile function can have an erection rigid enough for sexual intercourse.) That's the best-case scenario. If a tumor approaches the neurovascular bundle, a surgeon will remove it to improve the chance of eliminating all the cancer cells. Surgeons unfamiliar with the nerve-sparing approach, or who do not have the opportunity to perform it very often, generally aren't as successful at preserving potency. And older men, even in the care of expert surgeons, retain potency less often than younger men. Poor circulation, other complicating diseases like diabetes or emphysema, and even medication can contribute to loss of erections after a prostatectomy.

If erectile function is going to return, it will usually happen within twelve months to eighteen months. It can take that long for nerves and blood vessels to heal. Two years is probably the limit; beyond that it is unlikely that potency will return.

For all men, loss of potency can be an emotional, psychological, and physical blow. For those who were sexually active before surgery, it can be especially devastating. Fortunately, most men can still have an entirely pleasurable orgasm even without an erection. A prostatectomy does not damage the sensory nerves around the penis responsible for sexual pleasure, nor does it necessarily dampen a man's libido, his desire for sex. Some men adapt to this change and learn new ways to give and receive sexual pleasure with their partners. Others rely on one of several methods for inducing an erection, or opt for a penile implant that makes the penis rigid enough for intercourse (see Chapter 13).

INFERTILITY

As mentioned earlier, prostatectomy makes it impossible to father a child in the normal, time-honored manner, even if the operation doesn't affect the ability to have erections. During the operation the vas deferens is cut. This tube brings sperm from the testes to the urethra. In addition to the vasectomy, prostate removal causes dry ejaculations. Banking sperm before the operation and using it in one of several artificial-insemination techniques provides an option for the future.

BLEEDING
Like faces and physiques, internal anatomy varies from man to man. Blood vessels aren't always where the anatomy books say they are supposed to be. In the dim confines of the pelvis, some are nearly impossible to see and even harder to seal off. Postprostatectomy bleeding isn't uncommon; about 20 percent of men need a transfusion during the operation or recovery period. In most cases bleeding stops on its own. But when it is severe and does not gradually taper off, a trip back to the operating room to find and repair the leaky vessel is sometimes the only recourse.

ANASTOMOTIC LEAK
This is the name for a leak in the seal joining the two ends of the newly reconstructed urethra. Leaks usually appear soon after surgery, and are discovered when below-normal amounts of urine collect in the Foley catheter. Most heal spontaneously, but some anastomotic leaks must be repaired surgically. This means another trip to the operating room, where a surgeon opens you back up and stitches the ends of the urethra together more tightly.

ANASTOMOTIC STRICTURE
Scars form naturally whenever tissue is injured. Most of the time this disorganized growth rapidly seals a cut or scrape, reducing the chance of infection, like the abdominal scar you wear after a prostatectomy. A similar healing

process takes place in the urethra where the two ends were sewn together after the prostate was removed. If the new scar tissue takes up too much space or protrudes into the urethra, however, it can block urine flow. Strictures usually don't appear right away. In fact, it may take years for one to narrow the urethra enough to slow or block urination.

Strictures are usually treated by stretching or cutting the scar tissue. To do this a urologist inserts a thin, lubricated metal rod into the penis and gently works it into the urethra, past the stricture. Then he or she removes it and replaces it with another that's slightly wider. And another, and another until the stricture has been loosened. The procedure may have to be repeated several times over the course of a few months to effect a permanent change. Another way to open a stricture involves inserting a small scope into the urethra and cutting the scar tissue.

Rectal or Ureteral Tear

About 1 percent of all prostatectomies result in some injury to the rectal wall or the ureters, the tubes that carry urine from each kidney to the bladder. Removing the prostate can sometimes tear the rectum, because the two lie next to each other and may stick together. Or the rectal wall can be accidentally nicked with a scalpel during surgery. Such tears can lead to an infection of the abdominal cavity, and usually require surgery to repair. Damage to one or both ureters usually occurs when they enter the bladder in an unusual spot, just above the junction of prostate and bladder. Again, surgical repair is required.

Summing Up

The majority of postprostatectomy complications are unavoidable and unpreventable. They're neither your fault nor your surgeon's or nurses'. Remember, this is a major operation being done in a small, almost inaccessible cavity that is sometimes bathed in blood. If something happens that you didn't expect or weren't prepared for, talk to your physician. Ask him or her to explain what happened and how or why it occurred.

Keep in mind that all surgeons encounter complications, and the fact that one has occurred doesn't automatically mean he or she did anything wrong. The only reason for "firing" a surgeon is if you believe that it was his or her negligence that caused the complication. Otherwise, it makes sense to continue working with your original surgeon. He or she knows your case and your innermost anatomy and is in the best position to help you overcome the problem.

Cryosurgery

A semisurgical procedure that has been gaining a lot of media attention is called cryosurgery. It uses a supercold slush of liquid nitrogen to freeze the entire prostate gland, killing healthy and cancerous prostate tissue just as prolonged frostbite kills skin and muscle. While it has been used as treatment for tumors that persist after radiation therapy, some men are turning to cryosurgery as a primary treatment for small, gland-confined tumors (stages A and B). Swept aside by the hype that television, newspapers, and magazines accord any intriguing new medical technologies are some unanswered questions that you really should consider before opting for this procedure.

How It Is Done

One attractive feature of cryosurgery is that it requires no incisions. Instead, five probes the diameter of knitting needles are inserted into the prostate through the skin between the anus and scrotum—once you've been numbed with either a local or general anesthetic. The cryosurgeon uses a transrectal ultrasound machine to see each probe and position it precisely in the prostate. A special catheter is also inserted into the urethra. Once everything is in place, insulated hoses are attached to each probe and supercold liquid nitrogen is allowed to circulate through them. This literally turns the prostate into a ball of ice for a few minutes. Meanwhile, the urethra remains near body temperature thanks to the catheter, which has warm water circulating through it.

Recovery after the two-hour procedure is usually swift. Most men leave the hospital that day or the next, sporting a catheter to ensure urination and speed any urethral healing. It is usually removed after a few days. A week or so recuperating at home is generally sufficient before you can return to work or your regular activity, though it might be a bit longer before you should try strenuous exercise or labor.

Over the course of the next few months, white blood cells clean up the cellular debris left behind as prostate tissue dies. The prostate doesn't disappear, but turns into a slightly more compact nugget of scar tissue.

Side Effects

Side effects aren't as common after cryosurgery as they are after a radical prostatectomy. That's one of the advantages of this procedure. Since it doesn't require any incisions, there's little chance of an infection. And since you are back on your feet the next day, embolisms are rare. With the advent of the urethral warmer, incontinence due to urethral damage is also minimal with rates closer to those following radiation therapy than those following prostatectomy. Between 30 and 50 percent of men who were potent before cryosurgery can have an erection after the procedure—*unless* cryosurgery follows failed radiation therapy. Then the rates of all complications are dramatically higher.

An even more devastating side effect occurs in one to two men per 100 who have cryosurgery. The wall of the rectum, which sits only a few millimeters away from the prostate, sometimes freezes during the procedure. This can open a hole, or fistula, that can't always be surgically repaired. A man with a permanent fistula must excrete solid waste through an ostomy, an opening of the bowel permanently implanted on his abdomen.

Researchers know more about cryosurgery's side effects than they do about its long-term impact on prostate cancer. The first modern cryosurgeries were performed in 1990, and five years of follow-up just isn't enough time to tell if it will be an effective therapy. At Allegheny General Hospital in Pittsburgh, where modern cryosurgery was revived in 1990, at the University of California at San Diego, and at other institutions where this procedure has been used for several years, researchers talk in terms of "promising" negative biopsy rates at six months and one year. None has been able to evaluate whether this procedure prevents prostate cancer from spreading to other tissues or adds months or years to a man's life.

9

Radiation Therapy

(with Dr. William U. Shipley, Radiation Oncology)

High-energy radiation has played a central role in treating cancer since it was first suggested by Pierre Curie in 1910. A year later, French and Austrian physicians began inserting small radioactive "seeds" into cancerous prostate glands. Throughout the middle 1900s, cobalt-beam radiation was a mainstay in treating this disease. The introduction of hospital-sized linear accelerators in the late 1950s further refined this form of therapy. Today, roughly one-third of all men diagnosed with prostate cancer opt for radiation therapy.

The concept may sound like a contradiction in terms. After all, radiation from sources like an atom bomb or radon gas causes cancer. Yet it is radiation's very ability to kill or damage living cells, especially those that divide rapidly, that makes it a powerful weapon against some tumors. These include Hodgkin's disease, breast, testicular, and prostate cancer, among others.

Radiation therapy can be used to fight prostate cancer at several stages. It is appropriate for treating early-stage tumors confined to the gland—stage A (T1) and stage B (T2)—as are surgery and, in older men, watchful waiting. Radiation is sometimes used when a tumor appears to have escaped the gland and has begun growing in nearby tissue. Prostatectomy is usually not an option here because it is impossible for a surgeon to find, let alone remove, microscopic clumps of cells. Radiation can also be used to slow the spread of metastatic prostate cancer and ease the pain and symptoms that often accompany it. This chapter will focus on the first two. Its role in advanced prostate cancer is discussed in Chapter 12.

Advantages

Radiation has some distinct advantages:

• It requires no hospital stay or at-home recovery period, so it doesn't disrupt life as dramatically as surgery does. You continue to lead a fairly normal life that happens to be scheduled around daily therapy sessions.

• The immediate side effects are usually minor and controllable. There's no hair loss or severe nausea of the kind that accompanies radiotherapy for breast, brain, or lung cancer. A number of men suffer some fatigue, diarrhea, and bladder irritation, but these symptoms can often be blunted by some simple dietary tricks or medication.

• Incontinence isn't commonly associated with radiation therapy. For men who are continent before treatment, only 1 to 3 percent lose control of their urine stream following radiotherapy for prostate cancer. For the United States as a whole, the numbers for prostate surgery are significantly higher. At medical centers like Massachusetts General where hundreds of prostate surgeries are performed each year, loss of urinary control is about the same as with radiation therapy, though rates of stress incontinence are higher.

• It is as safe, if not safer, than surgery mostly because no potentially risky anesthesia is required. Nationally, the risk of dying from the side effects of radiation therapy is about one in 1,500 or more. By comparison, a recent review of Medicare records revealed that approximately one in 100 men die within three months of a prostatectomy, usually from a heart attack or stroke possibly triggered by the operation. For men over seventy, or those with other health problems, this number rises to eight in 100. (Again, the odds of dying during or soon after a prostatectomy are far lower at centers of excellence where surgeons routinely perform this demanding operation.)

Disadvantages

Radiation therapy also has its drawbacks:

• It requires a substantial time commitment that some men can't or don't want to make. The standard course of radiation for early-stage prostate cancer is one treatment per day, five days per week for seven to eight weeks. Each treatment takes an hour or less. Most radiation centers go out of their way to schedule appointments at convenient times, such as early in the morning, at the end of the working day, or during the lunch hour. Still, some men find it difficult to fit an hour-long radiation appointment into their schedules for thirty-five to forty consecutive working days. Men who live far from a medical center with modern radiotherapy equipment may also find the daily drive a burden.

• The prostate, its surroundings, and nearby lymph nodes never get the kind of direct scrutiny that surgery makes possible. Examining the removed prostate capsule or lymph nodes under the microscope can often tell if a tumor has spread beyond the gland or not, an important factor in planning treatment or predicting prognosis. In fact, 30 percent or more of men are "upstaged" after a prostatectomy, meaning their stage A (T1) or B (T2) cancer is reclassified to a stage C (T3) or D. A relatively new procedure called laparoscopic lymphadenectomy can circumvent this shortcoming of radiation therapy. A surgeon inserts a tiny camera and microscalpels or scissors through small punctures in the abdomen and removes a sampling of lymph nodes. This is similar to the "keyhole surgery" now routinely performed to remove a diseased gallbladder.

• Radiation therapy can't be repeated if the tumor recurs in the area around the prostate. A local recurrence of cancer after a prostatectomy can be treated with radiation or hormones. But only a few urologists in the United States recommend removing a previously irradiated prostate. This operation requires great surgical skill because radiation distorts the prostate and its surrounding tissues. It also makes these tissues fragile and difficult to operate on. In addition, previous radiation therapy compromises a tissue's ability to heal. Such so-called salvage prostatectomies are associated with very high rates of incontinence and other complications, and should only be performed by expert surgeons with plenty of experience in prostatectomies. Even more troubling, this procedure doesn't guarantee a cure, especially since by the time a man has this operation tumor cells may already have escaped the prostate (see page 229). The facts are these: 30 to 60 percent of those who have a salvage prostatectomy for what is thought to be cancer confined to the prostate are incontinent and virtually all are impotent. Five years down the line about 25 percent appear to be free of their cancer; however, five years is just not enough time to be sure the cancer will not recur. Some physicians believe that in the younger patient there may be a role for this type of surgery if done after radiation therapy when the PSA first begins to rise. In most cases, a recurrence of cancer following radiation leaves only hormone therapy in the armamentarium.

• About half the men who undergo radiation therapy for prostate cancer lose the ability to have erections within three years of treatment.

• Finally, men with a history of ulcerative colitis or prior bowel surgery usually don't tolerate radiotherapy very well.

As mentioned in previous chapters, the medical community is sharply divided over the roles of radiation therapy and surgery for early-stage prostate cancer. Some urologists claim that radiation therapy just isn't appropriate for men with stage A (T1) or stage B (T2) tumors. They believe radiation should be used only when surgery isn't an option, i.e., in cases where the tumor may have penetrated the prostate capsule, or if poor health makes a man a poor candidate for a prostatectomy. That is not, however, what a national panel of experts convened by the National Cancer Institute concluded in 1988:

Radical prostatectomy and radiation therapy are clearly effective forms of treatment in physicians' attempts to cure tumors limited to the prostate for appropriately selected patients. Comparisons across studies suggest comparable ten-year survival rates with either form of management. What remains unclear is the relative merit of each in producing lifelong freedom from cancer recurrence.[1]

Given such a strong statement, why this controversy? No valid study has ever directly compared the results of radiation therapy and prostatectomy against stage A (T1) or stage B (T2) prostate cancer. For scientists, the only way to prove if one technique is better than another requires what's called a prospective, randomized, controlled study. This would entail randomly assigning men with equivalent-stage tumors to either prostatectomy or radiation therapy and following how well they do over the next fifteen years. Given that most men would prefer the freedom to choose their own therapy, and the fact that research funding usually doesn't support such long-term studies, it is unlikely that such a study will ever take place.

So physicians try to compare results from prostatectomy studies with those from radiation studies. This is tougher than it sounds. Surgeons have the advantage of knowing exactly what stage cancer a man has, based on the pathology report. Radiation oncologists generally don't know if a tumor is confined to the prostate or has spread beyond it. Surgeons carefully select men who have the best chance of surviving a prostatectomy and benefiting from it, generally men whose tumors are confined to the gland and those with few complicating health problems. They usually refer to radiotherapy men whose tumors have likely spread beyond the prostate, men over

---

[1] National Institutes of Health, *Consensus Development Conference on the Management of Clinically Localized Prostate Cancer,* National Cancer Institute Monographs no. 7 (1988).

seventy or seventy-five, or men with "comorbidities" like heart disease, a previous stroke, severe diabetes, or other medical problems.

In other words, no one has been able to compare one group of men who chose radiation therapy with an identical group of men who had a prostatectomy. Unless the two populations differ in only one variable—the type of treatment—and everything else remains the same, comparing the results is like comparing bicycles with automobiles.

How It Works

The principle behind radiation therapy is simple: Bombarding a tissue with a beam of high-energy particles kills cells. These energetic particles knock electrons out of their atomic orbits, breaking chemical bonds right and left. What's left behind is a trail of highly reactive molecules that steal electrons from their neighbors, setting off a chain reaction that may take minutes or months to settle down. If the dose of radiation is small and the atoms affected aren't crucial, a cell can usually repair the damage. A similar chain of events occurs inside skin cells hit by ultraviolet radiation from the sun.

But a high dose of radiation, especially when it damages DNA—the complex chemical that makes human genes—can cause permanent damage. Slightly rearranging one small section of a DNA strand can rewrite a cell's genetic instructions and prevent it from carrying out important functions, stop it from replicating, or kill it outright.

The goal of radiation therapy is to destroy cancerous cells inside the prostate and in the zone of tissue surrounding the tumor. In doing so, healthy prostate cells are killed as well, turning the entire gland into a zone of nonfunctioning scar tissue. Blasting the prostate with a single, massive dose of radiation could achieve this effect. It would also irreparably damage important tissue near the prostate—the rectum, urethra, bladder, and intestines. The trick is to divide this single deadly dose into tolerable fractions and deliver it only to the prostate, missing nearby tissues. The most common radiotherapy regimen for prostate cancer today does just that. It takes thirty-five to forty hour-long visits—five a week for seven or eight weeks—to a medical center with a linear accelerator. (An experimental form of radiation therapy that uses small radioactive seeds implanted directly into the prostate is described later.)

Thirty-five visits seems like an awful lot; women with breast cancer often need only twenty treatments. "Many men are overwhelmed by the length of treatment," says MGH radiation oncology nurse Katie Mannix. "Some think it means their cancer is really bad, or worse than they had been told. It isn't. This strategy makes the treatment easier to tolerate and minimizes pain and inconvenience from side effects."

A linear accelerator (fig. 9.1) literally accelerates a beam of pure electrons—the tiny, negatively charged particles that revolve around atoms—until they are traveling at nearly the speed of light. Then it directs them at a small tungsten target, producing high-energy X rays that can be precisely focused on the prostate gland. Unlike lower-energy cobalt-based machines (which are no longer used to treat prostate cancer), a linear accelerator delivers radiation to the prostate without harming skin and other tissues that sit above or behind the gland. The older machines, used in the 1960s and 1970s, often caused in-

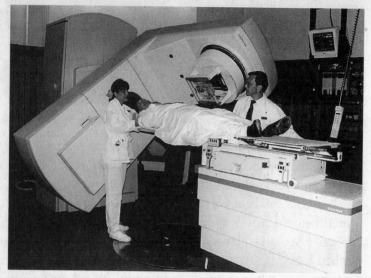

Figure 9.1. *The business end of a linear accelerator. A man lies on the treatment platform and the machine's rotating head precisely delivers high-energy radiation to the prostate gland.*

tense skin burns and tended to irradiate larger areas than needed. While the type of radiation generator is important, the experience and skill of the physician designing the treatment and prescribing the dose is crucial.

Radiation Therapy Procedure

"The key to successful radiation therapy is careful, careful planning," says Dr. William Shipley, MGH's chief of genitourinary radiation oncology. Knowing exactly where and how large the prostate is—it differs from man to man—makes it possible to accurately aim the radiation beam at the gland and minimize the chance of harming the bladder, rectum, or intestines. Mapping the prostate can be done several ways. Most centers use a treatment simulator, a room that looks exactly like the treatment room.

A radiation planning session at Massachusetts General Hospital takes one to two hours. It starts the same way almost every prostate-related test or checkup starts, with a rectal exam. The purpose of this one, however, is to locate the gland and guide the placement of two small slivers of gold. With one finger still in the rectum, the physician anesthetizes the skin between the scrotum and rectum with a shot of Novocain. Then he or she injects more Novocain deeper into the perineum, the tissue beneath that skin, stopping just short of the prostate. Once the perineum is numb, the physician inserts a long, thin needle through this area until it just touches the bottom of the prostate. Once in place, two gold nuggets smaller than chocolate jimmies are pushed out of the needle and into the prostate. They clearly appear on an X ray and unmistakably mark the very bottom of the gland.

Since the prostate fits snugly underneath the bladder, marking the bladder's bottom edge also marks the prostate's top. To do this, the physician lubricates the inside of the penis and inserts a catheter through the urethra and into the bladder. This procedure feels uncomfortable and may smart for a second or two, but after the catheter passes through the urethra you won't really feel it. Once in place, a small balloon on the catheter's tip is inflated, forming a plug that keeps it from sliding out of the bladder. A special contrast solution is poured into the bladder via the catheter. Both the inflatable tip and the solution show up on X rays, outlining the bladder and thus marking the prostate's top.

The third and final planning step takes place in the treatment simulator itself. You'll be asked to lie on a table that can move up, down, and sideways. A tube is placed in your anus, and your rectum filled with a dye that clearly shows up on an X ray. A series of X rays will be taken, each one followed by another table adjustment or two. Once the prostate is mapped and perfectly positioned under the linear accelerator's head, a technician places permanent ink dots on the skin over each of your hips and one on the pubis, just above your penis. These mark the spots where aligning laser beams touch the skin. This takes the guesswork out of proper positioning each treatment session. A technician merely adjusts the table so the dots line up with their respective laser beams and you're in the correct position. (If you notice these dots fading during your seven-week treatment, make sure to alert your physician or technician. Don't try to darken them yourself!)

That's it. Once the rectal tube and Foley catheters are removed, the planning session ends. Actual treatment sessions can begin in the next few days.

Each radiotherapy appointment takes roughly an hour—less than two minutes for the actual radiation, three to five minutes for positioning the table, and the inevitable waiting and searching for a parking space. You don't have to change into any special garb for the procedure, merely unbuckle your pants and lie on the table in your shorts. Once you've been lined up, the technician leaves the room. The invisible, unfelt radiation beam emanates from the head of the accelerator suspended over the table. Sometimes it stays in place, sometimes it rotates around the table. As soon as the daily fraction of radiation has been dispensed, the technician returns to the room, helps you off the table, and you're free to leave.

At no time during or after the procedure do you ever become radioactive. The linear accelerator hits you with short-lived, high-energy rays. Once they are trapped by tissue or body fluids, they lose their energy and settle down to become ordinary electrons. You won't set a Geiger counter to clicking, or glow in the dark. Feel free to pick up a grandchild, shake hands with a business associate, or make love with your partner. Nothing that comes out of you—saliva, urine, feces, semen, or sweat—is the least bit radioactive. (This only applies to external beam radiotherapy. Men with certain kinds of radioactive implants described later may need to stay in the hospital for a few days until the implants are removed or their radioactivity dissipates.)

Immediate Side Effects

During the first two or three weeks of therapy, few men notice any radiation-induced changes. Around week three or four, some begin to tire more easily or feel less energetic than usual. "It wasn't bad, but I noticed myself really dragging at the end of the day," says Tony, a seventy-one-year-old attorney.

The most common side effects during or immediately following radiation therapy include diarrhea and flatulence, burning upon urination, and the need to urinate more frequently than usual. About half of men experience one or more of these side effects, with loose bowel movements being the most common. Less common complications are rectal bleeding, pain during bowel movements, or urge incontinence. Nausea usually isn't a problem, as it is with radiation therapy for breast or lung cancer, since the beams don't go near the stomach.

These unpleasant effects occur because some radiation strikes the rectum, or hits the nearby bladder and intestines, on its way to the prostate. This irritates these muscular tissues and makes them prone to irregular spasms. In most cases these side effects disappear on their own within three weeks to three months after the last treatment session. In a small percentage of men, however, side effects persist longer than that.

Simple dietary changes can usually control diarrhea, flatulence, or painful defecation. The trick is making the intestines work as little as possible. Bland, processed foods like white bread, soda crackers, Cream of Wheat, and chicken are in; coffee is out, as is alcohol and spicy or un-processed foods like spareribs, tacos, beans, popcorn, onion, and garlic. In other words, you may have to give up many of the foods that make eating worthwhile, at least for a few weeks. Minimizing bladder irritation and uri-nary symptoms involves use of medications like the alpha-blockers used to control urinary symptoms stemming from benign prostatic hyperplasia.

Men receiving radiation therapy for prostate cancer at Massachusetts General Hospital get a list of simple tips for reducing gastrointestinal side effects, as well as a list of foods that MGH dietitians recommend and discourage. Going off your diet won't interfere with the effectiveness of treatment, but you may feel the aftermath. "I didn't re-ally stick to the bland diet I was supposed to stick to," says Bruce, a minister who needed radiation therapy after his prostatectomy at age fifty-five. "I'd eat barbecue or have a drink knowing full well that I would eventually pay the price for it with diarrhea or rectal burning."

About one in twenty men have severe enough side ef-fects that they need to stop radiation treatment for a week. Such an interruption doesn't make radiation treat-ment any less effective, points out Dr. Shipley.

Some simple tips for reducing diarrhea, gas, and urinary symptoms:

• Try to maintain your weight during treatment. "Some men actually gain weight when they stick to the diet we suggest and feel better for it," says Ms. Mannix.

• Soluble fiber absorbs water as it passes through the intestines and can dry up diarrhea. Stool-softening laxatives reduce the discomfort caused by normal or hard stools as they pass through an irritated rectum. Store brands include Metamucil or any generic product containing psyllium, as well as Fibercon or Citrucel.

• Eat a number of small meals during the day rather than two or three large ones. Avoid large first portions and skip second helpings. By doing this you give your intestines manageable amounts of food to process at any one time. Large meals make the intestines work harder; if they're irritated by irradiation they may not do the job as well as they should.

• To prevent bloating, limit the amount you drink with a meal to eight ounces. Between meals, drink noncarbonated beverages whenever possible.

• Take a supplement to make sure you are getting your daily requirement of vitamins and minerals. An inexpensive generic brand will do just fine.

• Switch from regular milk to one low in lactose, or milk sugar. Many adults have a tough time digesting lactose, and radiation can compound the problem. Low-lactose brands such as Lactaid or Dairy Ease can reduce gas and bloating.

• Cut back on your alcohol intake, since alcoholic beverages stimulate bowel and bladder activity, increasing both diarrhea and urinary symptoms. The occasional drink now and then won't be disastrous. "If you are used to having a drink before or with dinner, do it. It's important to maintain your normal lifestyle as close as possible," says Ms. Mannix.

Long-Term Side Effects

In a small proportion of men, the side effects that crop up during treatment persist for months or longer after that last session with the linear accelerator. One is rectal urgency, or the sensation that a bowel movement can't be held back for more than five or ten minutes. This uncommon side effect can be controlled with medication and generally fades away after a few months. Two others make themselves felt long after treatment has ended— impotence may appear anytime during the first one to five years, urethral or bladder-neck strictures can develop even later than that, as can episodes of bleeding in the urine or stool. And all men who have radiation therapy become infertile, even if they can still have erections (Fig. 9.2). As radiation therapy continues to get more and more precise, thanks to computer-assisted planning and CT scanning, the incidence of side effects should steadily decline.

Rectal Bleeding

No matter how carefully radiation therapy is planned or performed, it's very difficult to protect rectal tissue from harm. The rectum sits just below the prostate gland, with only a few millimeters of tissue separating the two. Radiation beams invariably penetrate the prostate and hit cells in the rectal lining. If these rapidly growing cells receive

Figure 9.2. Complications of radiation therapy in patients with tumors confined to the prostate

Number of patients	331
Deaths	0
Total incontinence	0.4%
Loss potency	63%
Diarrhea	
incidence	3.6%
persisting	0
GI strictures	
incidence	5.4%
persisting	1.2%
Hematuria	
incidence	5.1%
persisting	0.9%
Rectal bleeding	
incidence	5.4%
persisting	0.6%

SOURCE: *Journal of Urology* 1994, 152:1799

only small doses, then you'll probably experience only minor irritation during the seven-week procedure. But if your cells are especially sensitive to radiation or they receive a large enough accumulated dose of it, they begin dying off. This is occasionally accompanied by rectal bleeding. You might notice a reddish tinge to a bowel movement or two. Or you could see a bloody stripe on toilet tissue. Don't panic! This condition, sometimes called radiation proctitis, is more annoying than life-threatening. But report all rectal bleeding to your doctor so he or she can rule out other causes.

Rectal irritation can last for several months after radiation therapy ends. There's no single way to take care of it, though therapy generally includes a bland diet designed not to irritate the rectal walls. Time is one of the most important cures. Corticosteroids, often administered in suppository form, are sometimes used to decrease the inflammation.

Incontinence

Radiation can make the bladder highly irritable and spasmodic, especially in men who were prone to this condition prior to treatment. In a mild case, you feel as if you need to go to the bathroom even when the bladder contains little urine. Severely irritated bladders can cause urge incontinence, in which the urge to urinate comes on so suddenly and with such strength that a man can't hold it in until he finds a bathroom.

About 1 to 3 percent of men report some kind of incontinence following radiation therapy. In many, this means losing a few drops of urine during a sneeze or at times of physical exertion. Such stress incontinence can be controlled with Kegel exercises or by lining the underwear with a pad. But it can also be much worse and dramatically curtail a man's work, social life, physical activity, and sex life. A variety of methods for controlling moderate and severe incontinence are described in Chapter 13.

Stricture

Prostate irradiation can sometimes irritate the urethra or bowel so much that it scars or knots up, blocking the flow of urine or feces. This blockage, or narrowing, is called a stricture. A urologist can open most urethral strictures by slowly dilating them with a rounded probe inserted through the tip of the penis. This procedure is usually done under local anesthesia. Some strictures require surgery to cut the offending scar tissue and reseal the undamaged sections of urethra or bowel. Because the tissue had been previously irradiated, healing can take a long time and the seam doesn't always hold.

Impotence

When small arteries in the penis relax, they fill up with blood and cause an erection. The "on" switch is a signal from nerves that run from the spinal cord to the penis. Along the way they attach to the prostate capsule for support and protection. Radiation can damage these nerves and their associated blood vessels, though it often takes months for this damage to diminish or abolish a man's capacity for erections. In fact, few men lose their erections during the treatment period or the first few months afterward. One year later approximately 75 percent of men who were potent before radiation therapy can still get and maintain an erection. Five years later that number is down to 50 percent. While younger, healthy men are more likely to retain their erections, there's currently no accurate way to predict who will and who won't.

Radiation does not, however, damage the sensory nerves on the penis, nor does it affect the production of testosterone. In other words, men who can't have an erection after radiation therapy still have an interest in sex and the ability to have a normal, pleasurable orgasm. When faced with this kind of impotence, some men choose to give up sex altogether. Others experiment with their partner and learn new ways to give and receive sexual pleasure. Still others take advantage of new technology that can create erections, such as vacuum pumps, injections of drugs into the penis, or penile implants that are either permanently rigid or inflatable (see Chapter 13).

Infertility

In addition to killing tumor cells, radiation also kills normal prostate cells. So after radiotherapy the gland is no longer able to make or secrete the fluids needed to nourish and protect sperm. In other words, prostate irradiation makes a man infertile. For most men who develop prostate cancer, this isn't usually a concern. But if you harbor the hope of having a child or two, make sure you store some sperm before treatment. Ask your physician for a referral or look in the Yellow Pages under "sperm bank" or "infertility center."

After Treatment

When you walk out of the treatment center after your thirty-fifth or fortieth session, you're on your own for a while. Don't be surprised if a bit of sadness tinges the freedom and accomplishment you feel. "I got to feel very close with some of the other guys I would see every day while we were waiting for our turns on the machine," says Bob, a fifty-five-year-old publishing vice president who underwent radiotherapy after his prostatectomy turned up positive margins. "We traded a lot of information and almost formed a mini support group right there."

What follows treatment is an extended period of watching, waiting, and hoping all interwoven with getting on with your old life. During the first year, you will probably see your urologist every two or three months and your radiation oncologist every three to six months. These visits will involve a rectal exam and PSA test and should include plenty of time for you to ask any questions you have. Don't expect your PSA to immediately plummet to normal levels, as it would after surgery. Some of the cells injured by high-energy radiation take a year or more to die. Even as they fade away, they produce prostate-specific antigen and empty it into the bloodstream. What you hope for is that your PSA continues to drop from visit to visit, or at least remain stable. Some recently published research suggests that PSAs of 0.5 or lower are the best indicators that the cancer has been eradicated.

After the first year, your physician will probably suggest a PSA and rectal exam once every six months. Once you've successfully hit the five-year milestone, he or she will stretch out the time between visits to once a year. Don't skip these routine checkups, not even after five or ten years have passed. Prostate-cancer cells grow and divide so slowly that forming an identifiable tumor can take a decade. Men diagnosed with lung or testicular cancer who are still alive and disease-free five years after treatment can safely call themselves cured and not expect the disease to recur. Not so with prostate cancer. Recurrences can and do appear ten to fifteen years down the road.

Adjuvant Radiotherapy

Radiation therapy is recommended for some men who have just had prostate surgery. This double-barreled approach is used when the postprostatectomy pathology analysis finds cancer cells in the tissue surrounding the gland and a bone scan rules out the presence of distant metastases. Radiation to the prostate bed—the area where the prostate was embedded—may kill escaped cancer cells before they get the chance to grow and spread further. You may hear this called adjuvant radiotherapy, as opposed to primary radiotherapy. In the world of cancer treatment, *adjuvant* refers to a second form of therapy that boosts the success rate of the first one.

In terms of preparation and daily routine, adjuvant radiation does not differ from first-line radiation. Careful planning is needed to ensure that the high-energy beam strikes only the target area and not the entire pelvic region. And each day's visit takes about an hour—one to two minutes of actual treatment plus table arranging and the inevitable waiting time. It usually requires thirty sessions, compared to thirty-five to forty for primary radiotherapy.

Men who add radiation therapy after a prostatectomy with positive margins appear to do better than men who don't, though actual numbers won't be available for several years. Clinicians talk in terms of "disease-free survival rates." This is the proportion of men who remain free of prostate cancer after treatment, as measured by low or steady PSA levels. For men with positive margins who do not have adjuvant radiation, disease-free survival at five years is about 50 percent, meaning half have a steady PSA that indicates the absence of prostate cancer. For men who opt for adjuvant radiation therapy, five-year disease-free survival is about 66 percent, according to results from MGH and other centers.

Men undergoing adjuvant radiation therapy may be more likely to experience side effects, particularly incontinence. This is partly because the tissues receiving radiation have just been through a stressful operative procedure, which makes them less resilient and more prone to irritation. However, the same strategies used to minimize side effects in primary radiation therapy can be equally effective here.

Seed Implantation

Implanting tiny radioactive seeds, the first high-energy treatment ever tried for localized prostate cancer more than eighty years ago, is making something of a comeback. The idea makes great medical sense—radiation from the seeds strikes only the prostate, potentially reducing the side effects associated with radiation therapy.

Thanks to new technology, especially ultrasound and CT imaging, seed implantation may someday join external beam radiation and surgery as widely accepted therapies for cancer confined to the prostate gland—*if* long-term results live up to their early billing. CT scanning helps physicians make a three-D model of the prostate so they can carefully plan how many seeds are needed and where they should go. Ultrasound allows a physician to direct seeds to their appointed spots and hopefully ensure that the entire gland receives sufficient radiation.

Today, radioactive seed implantation does not require open surgery. Between fifty and eighty seeds are placed inside hollow needles (one seed per needle) which are pushed through the anesthetized skin between the scrotum and anus and into the prostate. An ultrasound probe in the rectum allows the physician to see exactly where each seed is placed. The procedure takes about two hours or so. Most men return home the same day, and quickly return to full activity. "I had my seeds put in on a Tuesday and was out for a hike in the woods on Saturday. I was back at work on Monday, though I sure wasn't ready to do any heavy lifting," says Hans, a sixty-six-year-old tax adviser.

Because the radiation is delivered slowly and continuously from the inside out, there may be less damage to nonprostate tissue and thus fewer rectal side effects than accompany external beam radiation. Diarrhea and rectal bleeding occur less frequently, and usually don't appear for two to four months. Urinary irritation, however, occurs with similar frequency. Nor is incontinence a problem, except in men who have already had a transurethral resection of the prostate (TURP) for benign prostatic hyperplasia. Seed implantation may cause less impotence than external beam radiation. For men under seventy about 65 percent of those who were potent before treatment maintain their ability to have erections; for men over seventy that number drops below 50 percent, according to radiation oncologist Dr. John Blasko of the Northwest Tumor Institute in Seattle, whose team has performed close to one thousand seed implants over the last ten years.

Everything about this technique sounds great—it is easy to perform, requires very little recovery, and doesn't have too many complications or side effects. The only thing missing is how it stacks up against external beam radiation or prostatectomy. And that information will remain missing for several more years. Published studies from Dr. Blasko and other researchers haven't been able to follow many men for very long periods. The average follow-up time is under four years—and almost every treatment strategy looks like a success over that short a period.

The bottom line is this: Seed implantation appears to be a promising technique, but at this point it is still a gamble.

Who's a candidate for this technique? Any man with a prostate-confined tumor (stage A or B) could take advantage of brachytherapy, just as he could external beam radiation or surgery. Large tumors or large prostate glands can pose a problem and may be better treated with external beam radiation. At first, seed implantation was recommended only for older men or those with other health problems, since the treatment causes relatively few side effects. As investigators hone their technique, a growing number of men are choosing this option simply because it makes sense to them.

10

Hormone Therapy

(with Dr. Donald S. Kaufman, Hematology/Oncology)

Throughout a man's life, the size and health of his prostate are intimately tied to hormones coursing through the bloodstream. As a Y-chromosome-bearing fetus develops, male hormones called androgens direct a small portion of the embryonic urinary and genital system to turn into the prostate. The surge of hormones that makes a teenage boy grow inches almost overnight, sprout pubic hair, and take a sudden interest in sex also triggers a period of explosive growth inside the prostate. During the teen years it more than quintuples in size, an amazing change when you consider that prostate cells are the body's growth and division slowpokes. During most men's fifties, sixties, and seventies, hormones again prompt prostate cells to grow and divide. This late-in-life growth spurt causes urinary problems that frustrate and irritate millions of men fifty and older (see Chapter 3).

Androgens, a type of steroid hormone, drive each of these changes. Testosterone is the most abundant androgen. It is commonly called the male hormone despite the fact that women's bodies also manufacture small amounts of it. Testosterone plays many different roles in a man's body. During fetal growth it directs development of male organs and body pattern. During adolescence it stimulates the growth of facial and body hair, deepens the voice, and prompts the sex organs to mature. Throughout adulthood, testosterone must be available for the testes to make sperm cells. It helps bone marrow generate red blood cells and is needed to build muscle. It somehow sparks the libido, or desire for sex. And last but not least, testosterone controls the growth of prostate cells. Men who for one reason or another can't manufacture this hormone never suffer from benign prostate enlargement.

Since prostate-cancer cells arise from normal prostate cells, they too have an affinity for testosterone. While not an absolute requirement for tumor-cell growth and division, this hormone is high on the list of necessary substances. Think of it as fertilizer. Unfortunately, merely withholding this fertilizer won't kill off prostate cancer cells any more than this trick kills off crabgrass and weeds in your yard. Normal levels of testosterone encourage growth of these cells while its absence curbs, but doesn't necessarily arrest, their growth, division, or spread.

The connection between testosterone and prostate cancer was suspected two centuries ago. But it took a University of Chicago surgeon to firmly establish the connection. In the early 1940s, Dr. Charles Brenton Huggins removed the testes, where testosterone is manufactured, from a number of men with advanced prostate cancer. In almost every case, castration shrank their tumors, reduced their pain, and lengthened survival by months or years. For figuring out how hormones influence prostate cancer, Huggins was awarded the 1966 Nobel Prize in medicine and physiology. Today, variations of his approach are a mainstay of prostate-cancer treatment, especially when the tumor has escaped from the gland.

Hormone therapy, unlike surgery or radiation, does not remove, inactivate, or kill tumor cells. Instead, it cuts off the supply of testosterone and figuratively starves these cells into hibernation. Unfortunately, most prostate-cancer tumors eventually adapt to low testosterone levels and begin to grow and divide without needing a hormone signal. For this reason, hormone therapy is never used as a *cure* for prostate cancer. Instead, it is used to hold the disease at bay, temporarily shrinking tumors that strangle the urethra, block the kidneys, or press on nerves in the spinal cord. It can also delay the inevitable spread of advanced prostate cancer. In the anticancer armamentarium, hormone therapy offers the only effective defense against disease that has spread beyond the prostate or metastasized to other parts of the body.

No one knows exactly why hormone therapy eventually stops working. The average prostate tumor probably starts its life from a single renegade cell. As that one cell becomes billions, small genetic errors crop up and are passed along. Over time, some of these mutant cells acquire the ability to live and grow without a testosterone signal. Once the hormone-dependent cells have been deprived of testosterone and stunned into inactivity, these others seize the opportunity to proliferate and gradually take over. No matter what the mechanism, hormone therapy invariably loses its ability to keep tumor cells in check. In most men this occurs within one to five years; for some lucky ones hormone therapy can work for a decade or more.

Even though hormone therapy has been used against late-stage prostate cancer for half a century, new advances and techniques are raising some controversy. So far, there's no rock-solid agreement among the experts when it comes to:

- Who should get hormone therapy: Traditionally used for men with stage D prostate cancer, it is now being prescribed for men with stage A (T1) through stage D. Some researchers use it in conjunction with radical prostatectomy or radiation therapy, when it is called adjuvant therapy.
- When to begin hormone treatment: In the not-too-distant past, hormone therapy was started when symptoms such as bone pain or kidney blockage indicated that prostate cancer had spread beyond the gland. Today, bone scans and PSA tests can identify tumor metastasis long before it engenders any symptoms. Some physicians recommend beginning hormone therapy once symptoms appear; others encourage men to start it well before they suffer any symptoms. Both approaches have benefits and drawbacks.
- The best method of eliminating or blocking testosterone: The choices include surgical castration, a host of different drug regimens that are the medical equivalent of castration, and total androgen ablation—stopping androgen production by the adrenal glands as well as the testes.

The sections below describe how hormone therapy works, the different methods of hormone therapy, and the advantages and drawbacks of each.

How It Works

Testosterone acts like a traffic signal for prostate and prostate-cancer growth. When molecules of this hormone enter the gland via the bloodstream, they essentially give prostate-cancer cells the green light to grow and divide. Their absence brings this activity to a screeching halt, though some very aggressive cells can run the red light.

Special cells in the testes convert cholesterol—that nasty fat we're supposed to eat in very limited quantities—into testosterone. The average man makes approximately six milligrams of testosterone a day. Over the course of a year that amounts to slightly more than two grams, about what a penny weighs. Blood flowing through vessels in and around the testes pick up this hormone and carry it throughout the body. The normal range for testosterone in a blood sample is between 300 and 1,100 nanograms per deciliter of blood. (You'll see this written in a medical chart as ng/dl.) Much of this testosterone is bound to a carrier or transport protein called sex-hormone-binding globulin; only about 5 percent of it wanders freely in the blood.

The testes don't churn out the same amount of testosterone every hour of every day. Instead, they follow a daily cycle that usually peaks in the morning and hits bottom at night. They also respond to demand much the same way a thermostat responds to room temperature. When blood testosterone levels fall below some set point, a signal from the body turns on the testosterone-making machinery. As the testosterone in the bloodstream rises, production slows, then ceases altogether when levels creep above the set point.

The testosterone thermostat sits in a tiny knob of the brain called the hypothalamus, situated directly behind the bridge of the nose. It monitors and controls rhythmic body functions like hunger, thirst, sleep, and reproductive function. When the hypothalamus senses low testosterone levels, it secretes a protein called luteinizing-hormone-releasing hormone (LHRH) into the bloodstream (fig. 10.1). Cells in the pituitary gland, conveniently snuggled underneath the hypothalamus, absorb LHRH and begin secreting another protein called luteinizing hormone (LH) into the bloodstream. Once in the testes, luteinizing hormone stimulates a group of cells to make testosterone. High testosterone levels, in turn, act directly on the hypothalamus to shut off LHRH secretion. No LHRH means no more LH secreted by the pituitary, and thus no more

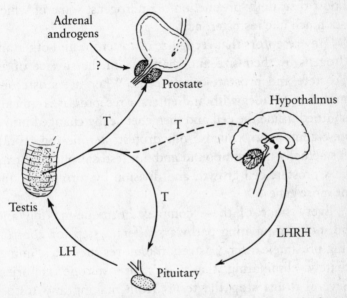

Figure 10.1. *One of a man's many hormonal cycles. The hypothalamus produces luteinizing hormone releasing hormone (LHRH), which stimulates the pituitary gland to produce luteinizing hormone (LH). Once in the bloodstream, LH stimulates the testicles to produce testosterone (T). Testosterone not only acts on the prostate, but also makes the hypothalamus stop producing LHRH. Hormones produced by the adrenal glands may also affect the prostate.*

testosterone production. This complex cycle certainly violates engineering's KISS (Keep It Simple, Stupid) principle. Biologically, however, it makes perfect sense, offering several spots for exquisite control and feedback.

The remaining players in this cycle are the adrenal glands. Perched atop each kidney, they secrete about 10 percent of the total daily production of androgens (about 5 percent of daily testosterone). Once the testes have been removed or their testosterone-making cells shut down, however, feedback signals stimulate the adrenal glands to boost their daily production of androgens, some of which act much like testosterone.

Tiny receptors that recognize testosterone and other androgens by their size and shape sit on the surface of all prostate and prostate-cancer cells. When a testosterone molecule collides with and enters a receptor, it is quickly shuttled inside the cell and then chemically changed into a new compound, called 5-dihydrotestosterone (fig. 10.2). It's actually this compound and not testosterone that triggers prostate-cell growth and division by turning on one or more genes.

Every stage of these complex hormone-making and hormone-stimulating pathways offers a step for controlling prostate cancer. Castration removes the testes, immediately eliminating the body's testosterone factories. Several drugs stop the testes from making any testosterone, offering a form of medical castration. Others prevent prostate-cancer cells from recognizing testosterone in the bloodstream. Still others block their ability to convert testosterone into 5-dihydrotestosterone.

In theory, depriving prostate-cancer cells of a steady supply of testosterone halts their growth, division, and spread. In practice, however, it's never that simple. Be-

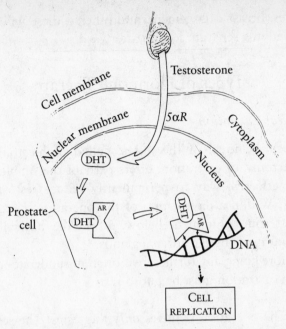

Figure 10.2. *Inside a prostate or prostate cancer cell, testosterone is converted into dihydrotestosterone (DHT) by an enzyme called 5-alpha reductase. The dihydrotestosterone joins up with a protein receptor (AR), and together they signal the cell's genetic material—and thus the cell itself—to replicate and divide.*

tween 10 and 20 percent of men with prostate cancer have a tumor that can grow even in the absence of testosterone and other androgens. As mentioned earlier, tumors that *are* dependent on testosterone don't stay that way permanently. Over time they gradually acquire the ability to grow and divide without a hormone signal.

The most common types of hormone therapy are described below. Since they share the same constellation of side effects—impotence, shrinking libido or sex drive, hot flashes, breast enlargement, and others—these will be explained in a separate section afterward.

Types of Hormone Therapy

Surgical Castration

Surgical removal of the testes, called orchiectomy, orchidectomy, or castration, offers perhaps the simplest and most effective way to permanently reduce testosterone levels. Within a day or two of the operation, circulating testosterone plummets below 50 ng/dl, basically the amount made by the adrenal glands.

Before going any further, two often misunderstood facts about castration must be put to rest:

• The operation removes *only* the testes. The scrotum and penis remain intact. Even in a well-lit locker room, it's virtually impossible for anyone to tell if a man has had an orchiectomy.

• Removing the testes won't change the way a man looks, sounds, or acts. A deep voice won't rise, nor a beard disappear or balding accelerate.[1] Castration won't make a man sexually interested in other men. In fact, it will most likely snuff out his desire for sex.

Castration effectively and irreversibly reduces testosterone levels. Between 70 and 90 percent of men with symptoms of advanced prostate cancer respond to this

---

[1] A few men on combination hormone therapy report a regrowth of fuzz atop previously bald pates. The treatment probably won't ever challenge minoxidil (Rogaine) in the marketplace—not too many men would trade the ability to have erections and an interest in sex for a full head of hair!

treatment within a week or so. Tumors pressing on the urethra or nerves shrink, improving urination and relieving pain. The beneficial effects last, on average, one to two years for men with advanced stage D tumors. Some men, however, survive for many years. In general, the less tumor present throughout the body the longer hormone therapy will prolong survival.

An orchiectomy takes only an hour to perform, and most men go home from the hospital the same day. It can be done under local anesthesia, though most men prefer to sleep through the procedure. The surgeon opens the scrotum with an incision down the midline, revealing the testes. He or she cuts the two spermatic cords, one above each testis, which frees the two egg-shaped glands. The spermatic cords, which contain the vas deferens, nerves, and blood vessels, remain in the scrotum. Some men opt to have one or two prosthetic testes placed in the scrotal sac at this time, or in a separate procedure several months later. I usually suggest to my patients that they wait and see what happens. It's quite easy to curl the cords up inside the scrotum during the operation so it looks and feels as if the testicles are still there. That often gives a man the physical confidence and peace of mind he needs without implanting a foreign object that can break or get infected.

Few complications ordinarily follow an orchiectomy. Bleeding from the spermatic cords can cause the scrotum to swell a little, but this usually goes down by itself over a week or two. Pain is minimal and of the kind that can be kept in check with Tylenol or some other over-the-counter painkiller, as long as it doesn't contain aspirin. (Aspirin inhibits clotting and can prolong any internal bleeding.) As with any operation, infections can crop up. Any postsurgery fever, excessive swelling, bruising, or reddening of the incision should be brought to your surgeon's attention.

Medical Castration

Researchers have devised several ways to throw a medical monkey wrench into the testosterone-making machinery. A variety of drugs stop the brain from making luteinizing hormone, the hormone that tells the testes to make more testosterone. Others inactivate testosterone-making cells in the testes and adrenal glands. Still others block prostate-cancer cells from recognizing testosterone or grabbing it from the bloodstream.

Some of these drugs are as effective as surgical castration. All, however, ultimately cost more than an orchiectomy, require daily or monthly attention and regular physician visits, and can lead to more disturbing side effects. Despite these drawbacks, about 70 percent of men who need hormone therapy choose the medical route over surgery.

LHRH AGONISTS
Compounds called LHRH agonists mimic the size and shape of luteinizing-hormone-releasing hormone, the molecule that starts the cascade of reactions leading to testosterone production. Examples of LHRH agonists include leuprolide (Lupron), goserelin (Zoladex), and buserelin. So far, only Lupron has the Food and Drug Administration's stamp of approval for use in the United States. The others are available to men who participate in controlled clinical trials, mostly sponsored by the National Cancer Institute.

These drugs work by flooding LHRH receptors on the surface of pituitary gland cells, making the pituitary pump out LH nonstop and in much larger quantities than it's used to. After a few days, the exhausted pituitary begins absorbing LHRH receptors from its surface and shutting down LH production. The upshot of this is that testosterone levels skyrocket for a few days, then, as the LH supply dwindles, they fall to castration levels.

The side effects are essentially those encountered after an orchiectomy, described below.

During the first few weeks of therapy with Lupron or another LHRH agonist, testosterone levels surge before they permanently plunge. This "hormone flare" can suddenly enlarge tumors, a potentially dangerous situation. Rapid growth of a tumor pressing on the spinal cord can lead to severe pain or temporary paralysis, while rapid tumor growth around the urethra can suddenly block urine flow. To prevent this flare, an LHRH agonist is usually combined with an antiandrogen (see below) such as flutamide (Eulexin), nilutamide (Anandron), or bicalutamide (Casodex) for at least the first few weeks of therapy. These agents block testosterone's effects and thus blunt any symptom flare.

ESTROGEN THERAPY

The earliest form of medical hormone therapy for prostate cancer used estrogen, the female hormone. In a man, natural or synthetic estrogen has the same effect on the hypothalamus as testosterone does—it shuts off LHRH secretion. No LHRH means that the pituitary won't secrete any more LH. And no LH puts the brakes on testosterone production.

Research in the 1960s and 1970s, especially several large studies sponsored by the U.S. Veterans Administration, showed that daily doses of estrogen taken by men with stage D prostate cancer were as effective as castration at controlling local symptoms and stalling the spread of metastatic disease. As with other hormone therapies, however, it did not increase the average length of time that the men lived. But at the high doses used in these studies— five milligrams/day, the equivalent of eight birth-control pills—an alarming number of men died from heart attacks and stroke. Further studies showed that one milligram of estrogen daily was equally effective and substantially reduced the risk of cardiovascular complications.

Estrogen is easy to take and relatively cheap—a pill a day, costing about $400 a year. But because of its side effects, it may not be appropriate for you if you have a family or personal history of high blood pressure, stroke, or heart disease. If you do take estrogen for hormone therapy, report suspicious leg or chest pains to your physician immediately.

Other Methods of Hormone Therapy

While the majority of hormone therapies aim to reduce testosterone production, several other approaches exist. They can be used in combination with castration or an LHRH agonist or as stand-alone therapies. These other options can prove invaluable for men who don't respond to medical or surgical castration or who suffer from their side effects. They may also provide relief for men whose prostate or metastatic tumors have adapted to growing in the absence of testosterone.

ANTIANDROGENS
Several compounds have been discovered or developed that essentially blanket prostate and prostate-cancer cells

with a protective coat that prevents testosterone and other androgens from getting inside. Examples include flutamide (Eulexin), nilutamide (Anandron), and bicalutamide (Casodex.) These are described more fully below. Their solo use as first-line hormone therapy is still experimental. Most are used in concert with castration or an LHRH agonist to provide a complete hormone blockade. Megesterol acetate (Megace) and cyproterone acetate (Cytadren) are two synthetic steroid-type drugs that can sometimes be used as antiandrogens.

KETOCONAZOLE

This compound, originally used to fight fungal infections, works directly on the testes and adrenal glands to quell testosterone production. It stops testosterone production immediately, and can provide relief within a day for men with cancerous blockage of the urethra or kidneys, or severe pain from a tumor pressing on the spinal cord or other nerves. Since ketoconazole causes liver damage if used for too long, it is generally recommended only in emergencies.

Side Effects

The body doesn't passively accept turning off the testosterone pumps. It responds in a variety of ways, none of them pleasant but none of them deadly or life-threatening, either. Consequences of disrupting the normal hormone cycle can include impotence, loss of libido, hot flashes, breast enlargement, and loss of energy. Fixes exist for each of these if, or when, they become too irritating to live with or reduce the enjoyment a man gets from life.

Impotence and Sex Drive

Believe it or not, your interest in sex stems partly from a chemical. A man's brain is wired in such a way that sexual thoughts, fantasies, and the desire to make love or masturbate depend in large part on the presence of testosterone. This doesn't mean that men with a lot of testosterone are sexier or better lovers than men with low levels. But when testosterone virtually disappears from circulation, spontaneous or stimulated erections also disappear. The ability to feel sexual pleasure and the capacity for orgasm still remain, however.

Some men adapt to this change by giving up sex altogether. Others explore with their partner different methods of giving and receiving pleasure that don't focus on genital lovemaking. Still others turn to the drugs, devices, and implants described in Chapter 13.

Hot Flashes

More than half of men using some form of hormone therapy experience the same kind of hot flashes that plague most women going through menopause. These bursts of internal heat arrive without warning three, four, five, ten, or more times a day. They can strike while loading boxes, writing a report, taking a stroll, or sitting quietly. For some men, they disappear over a year or so. Others see no slowdown. These hot flashes can be chilled out several ways. A single estrogen or megesterol acetate pill every day can do the trick. The drug clomipramine, delivered via a patch worn on the skin, also works.

Breast Enlargement

Another common response to hormone therapy, this one embarrasses more than it irritates. One effective preventive treatment involves a short dose of radiation to each breast, which effectively stops cell division. The dose used doesn't make the breasts radioactive or cause breast cancer. But it may be a more aggressive therapy than some men want to pursue for this condition.

Loss of Muscle Mass

Weight-lifters, football players, and other athletes sometimes take steroid hormones to quickly build muscle. Most of these are synthetic versions of testosterone, or closely related to it. So shutting off testosterone production also eliminates a compound needed to keep muscle tissue healthy and growing. Men on hormone therapy for several years can see their muscles shrink and weaken. Exercise that includes some kind of arm- and leg-weight training can help preserve the muscles you have and keep them strong.

Fatigue

A kind of cumulative fatigue accompanies long-term hormone therapy. "It's not really noticeable at first, and creeps up on you little by little," says Barry, a seventy-three-year-old former police officer. There aren't many antidotes. Get as much sleep as you need. Rest when you're tired. Try some gentle exercises like a walk around the block. Drink a cup of coffee or tea. "Basically, you just have to adjust," he suggests.

Combined Hormone Therapy

Medical or surgical castration doesn't completely dry up the supply of male hormones in the body. After an orchiectomy, testosterone levels in the bloodstream drop by 95 percent or more. But inside the prostate, levels of its highly active cousin, 5-dihydrotestosterone, drop by only 60 percent or so, thanks to androgens produced by the adrenal glands.

As might be expected, falling testosterone levels rev up androgen secretion by the adrenal glands. Some androgens are eventually changed into testosterone, others find their way into prostate and prostate-cancer cells where they are converted into 5-dihydrotestosterone. The net result is that adrenal-generated androgens may have an impact on prostate-cancer growth. Removing the adrenal glands isn't an option, since they also produce essential hormones that regulate energy metabolism and blood pressure.

The adrenal glands respond to a different set of signals from the pituitary and testes. They don't recognize LHRH and LH, or use them to trigger androgen production. So traditional hormone therapy leaves the adrenal's hormone-making machinery intact and working faster than normal, pumping out a small but steady supply of potential prostate-cancer fertilizer.

The Antiandrogens

Drugs called antiandrogens can protect prostate-cancer cells against this residual testosterone. These compounds have the same size and shape as testosterone and other androgens. Like poorly duplicated keys, they fit into lock-like androgen receptors on the surfaces of prostate and prostate-cancer cells. But once inside the receptor they stay jammed in place, making it impossible for circulating testosterone or other androgens to get inside the cell. The antiandrogen most commonly used in the United States is flutamide (Eulexin). That's because it has been approved by the Food and Drug Administration for several years. After several years of intensive testing, bicalutamide (Casodex) was approved in November 1995. Nilutamide (Anandron) is widely used in Europe but not yet approved for use in the United States.

Although the concept of total androgen blockade makes great theoretical sense, there is intense controversy in the medical community over whether it is either necessary or helpful in men whose testosterone levels are down to so-called castrate levels. Ongoing clinical trials aimed at clearing up this controversy won't have any practical answers for several more years.

FLUTAMIDE

You take two flutamide pills every eight hours. *Caution*: This doesn't mean three times a day, or at each meal. Since the body breaks down antiandrogens as they circulate, you have to take these pills on schedule—say at 7:00 A.M., 3:00 P.M., and 11:00 P.M. Stretching the period between doses to ten and twelve hours allows androgens to intermittently sneak into prostate-cancer cells and keep them in growth mode. Most men tolerate this drug well, but about 10 to 20 percent experience negative side effects. The most common are diarrhea, breast enlargement, and skin rash. Some men report feeling depressed while on the drug, though this may be a combination of drug therapy and the emotional turmoil that surrounds having and fighting cancer.

Bicalutamide

This compound works just like flutamide. But it has one difference that could be a boon to men who need an antiandrogen: Casodex lasts longer in the body and needs to be taken only once a day.

Nilutamide

Like flutamide, this drug is taken in pill form three times a day and the same warning applies to it. Roughly 90 percent of men who take nilutamide have trouble seeing at night, because the drug somehow interferes with the eyes' ability to adjust to darkness after looking at a bright light. This can be a real problem when driving. Normal dark adaptation returns soon after stopping the drug. Nilutamide also predisposes men to developing a lung disease called interstitial pneumonitis.

Does Combined Hormone Therapy Work?

Medical research hasn't yet determined if combined hormone therapy—taking daily antiandrogen pills after an orchiectomy or in concert with monthly LHRH-agonist injections—is worth the physical and monetary cost. Some studies show it offers little benefit; others show a clear advantage. Sometimes a single study has been interpreted both ways. Take an important 1989 trial sponsored by the National Cancer Institute that followed men with advanced stage D2 tumors. Those who took leuprolide plus flutamide (Lupron plus Eulexin) fared better than men taking leuprolide plus a placebo, or sugar pill. Median survival—the point at which 50 percent of the men in each group were alive and 50 percent had died—was thirty-five months for the combination and twenty-nine months for the leuprolide alone. A closer look at the data revealed even more encouraging news. For men with "minimal" metastatic disease, meaning relatively low PSAs and fewer than five sites of bone metastasis, median survival was sixty-one months for the combination therapy and forty-one months in the leuprolide-only group.

Critics challenge the conclusion that the combination therapy prolongs life. They offer an alternative, equally plausible explanation: The men on leuprolide alone suffered from the "flare phenomenon" that is now known to initially accompany use of an LHRH agonist. During this three- or four-week period, testosterone levels spike upward before the testes stop making it. This temporarily stimulates tumor growth and may make symptoms flare up. Even a brief period of permissive tumor growth could have diminished the survival of men taking leuprolide alone. Had one group of men in the study taken flutamide only through the flare period, then continued with leuprolide alone, these critics argue, they would have lived as long as those who took the leuprolide-flutamide combination for years.

Today, most men who opt for a medical castration take flutamide or another antiandrogen along with an LHRH agonist for the first two months or so. Whether it makes sense to continue the combination beyond that point has yet to be proven. Clinical trials aimed at answering this pressing question are under way, but an answer won't be forthcoming for several years.

On the basis of the NCI work and other studies, especially those of Dr. Fernand Labrie and his associates at Laval University in Quebec, the national prostate-cancer support group called Patient Advocates for Advanced Cancer Treatment (PAACT) argues that combined hormone therapy is the *only* treatment a man should consider as his first step against advanced disease. PAACT founder Lloyd Ney passionately promotes this therapy, and with good reason—he's lived more than ten years since he was diagnosed with advanced prostate cancer. He attributes his survival to CHT and believes it would benefit other men as well. Mr. Ney deserves a lot of credit for his tireless work on behalf of men with prostate cancer and for his efforts to give them the best information available about treating this vexing disease. But one man's story, or even one hundred men's stories, of long-term survival doesn't offer a realistic picture. For every one of them, there are many others who died within a year or so of starting combined hormone therapy. Right now the numbers just aren't there to prove or disprove CHT's effectiveness.

PAACT even goes a giant step further and argues, sometimes quite stridently, that men with stage A and stage B prostate cancer should follow a four-month regimen of CHT before undergoing a radical prostatectomy or beginning radiation therapy. Surgical and radiation researchers around North America and Europe have been testing this concept for several years, but it is still too early to tell if it works or to discover any unsuspected hazards that may accompany this approach.

Timing of Hormone Therapy

In the days before PSA tests, a man and his physician knew it was time to begin hormone therapy when symptoms of advanced or metastatic prostate cancer appeared—bone pain, suspicious areas on a bone scan, urinary obstruction, or kidney blockage. Things aren't that straightforward today. A rising PSA after radiation therapy or a prostatectomy can pinpoint recurrent disease years before any symptoms occur. Some men and their physicians choose to start hormone therapy at this first telltale signal in the hopes that early treatment will slow the growth and spread of any remaining tumor cells.

According to Dr. Labrie, "Endocrine therapy for metastatic prostate cancer should be started as soon as a diagnosis of stage D2 prostate cancer is made. Such a strategy can add years and quality of life to prostate cancer patients."

Unfortunately, there's little hard evidence to support this approach. Most studies show that early hormone therapy increases something called disease-free survival, the period from diagnosis to the emergence of symptoms. It does not, however, appear to add any time to overall survival. Nor does this approach leave any effective weapons in the arsenal once symptoms do appear.

How to Choose

The lack of a clear consensus on both combined hormone therapy and early hormone therapy leave men asking: If CHT *might* work better than single therapy, and starting early *may* have an advantage over starting later, why shouldn't I try early CHT just for insurance? That's a good question. Early and combined hormone therapy certainly aren't any worse than their counterparts. So choosing them may make sense—once you've considered the drawbacks.

Remember, hormone therapy, whether it is accomplished by an orchiectomy or through drugs, invariably causes impotence and loss of libido. In the absence of symptoms, some men decline early hormone therapy in order to maintain a normal sex life as long as possible. Other side effects may also influence your choice. Hormone therapy often leaves a man feeling chronically tired or fatigued, which can limit activity. The low testosterone and estrogen levels that result from hormone therapy cause hot flashes. While they aren't the least bit harmful or life-threatening, some men find them particularly aggravating and unsettling. It can also cause breasts to swell or enlarge, a condition called gynecomastia. The antiandrogen flutamide irritates the stomach and causes diarrhea in 10 percent or more of men who take it. Nilutamide, another antiandrogen, causes night blindness in 90 percent or so of the men who take it, posing a problem for those who must drive or work at night.

Although the medical fixes described earlier can take care of these problems, some men just don't want to deal with them, especially if the treatment that causes them doesn't offer a clear benefit. Then there's the hassle factor. In order for combination therapy to work effectively, you must take the antiandrogen flutamide every eight hours. Not just three times a day, or with meals, but strictly every eight hours.

Finally, as mentioned earlier, hormone therapy can be costly. If your insurance covers the cost of drugs, then this isn't an issue. If it doesn't, combination hormone therapy with Lupron and Eulexin will set you back somewhere around $7,000 per year for the rest of your life. (Several pharmaceutical companies have assistance programs that offer expensive anticancer drugs to men at low or no cost. If your physician isn't familiar with such programs, write or call the drug companies directly. Or you can get information from PAACT or Us-Too.)

In the absence of a consensus, your own preferences should guide your decisions about hormone therapy. Some men need to stay in control by constantly and actively fighting prostate cancer. If you are like this, the peace of mind that early hormone therapy might bring is worth any side effects. If an active sex life is important to you and you don't mind the uncertainty of waiting for symptoms to appear, delaying hormone therapy can give you several side-effect-free years.

Perhaps one of the smartest things you can do is to talk with some men who have already made this decision. Call a local prostate-cancer support group and explain your problem. Odds are you will be put in touch with several others who have been down that road and whose experiences may help you.

Adjuvant Hormone Therapy

In medical lingo, an adjuvant is something that improves a drug's activity or a procedure's effectiveness. Hormone therapy is sometimes used as an adjuvant with surgery or radiation. This approach, while still experimental and not yet FDA-approved, is becoming more common across the United States.

Reducing the amount of testosterone in circulation shrinks tumors at least 70 percent of the time. The smaller a tumor, researchers reason, the more likely it will be confined to the prostate and thus easier to destroy with radiation or remove during surgery. Pretreatment hormone therapy could also kill off cells that may have escaped a small tumor and taken up residence elsewhere.

When hormone therapy is begun before surgery or radiation, it is sometimes called neoadjuvant hormone therapy. It usually entails taking an LHRH agonist like leuprolide for three or four months. An antiandrogen like flutamide or bicalutamide may also be part of the package. The goal is to see PSA levels drop by 80 percent or more before starting definitive treatment.

This is still an experimental approach. In most cases it is available only as part of a controlled clinical trial, although some urologists and radiation oncologists around the country who aren't affiliated with a clinical trial probably offer it as an option.

11

Watchful Waiting

Most of us associate cancer with action. Battle metaphors usually spring to mind: We talk about the war against cancer, fighting tumors with surgery, or bombarding them with radiation. A less aggressive technique that more closely resembles vigilant spying is gradually being tried against different cancers. This strategy, formally called watchful waiting or expectant management, monitors a tumor's growth without treatment and thus without the side effects of treatment.

Suicidal? Not when it comes to prostate cancer. Lung, liver, and other tumors demand immediate therapy since they grow so quickly and spread so rapidly throughout the body. Within six months of a diagnosis of pancreatic cancer, at least half of its victims have died. The best hope of curing or halting such fast cancers rests on catching them early and destroying them before they spread. The treatments needed to accomplish this often devastate the entire body, but people are usually willing to withstand side effects such as nausea, hair loss, fatigue, infection, and the risk of anesthesia and surgery because they are generally less severe than the ultimate result of unchecked tumor growth—death.

With prostate cancer, things aren't so clear-cut. Most prostate tumors *don't* grow quickly or spread like wildfire. Just the opposite. Small, well-differentiated tumors (Gleason sum 4 or less) grow more slowly than almost any kind of cancer known and usually remain in the prostate rather than disperse through the body. Even larger, poorly differentiated prostate tumors aren't nearly as aggressive as most fast cancers. This slow growth gives some men with prostate cancer the opportunity to merely monitor their tumor and defer action for years.

Doing nothing against prostate cancer sounds crazy. But for some men it makes perfect sense. This disease usually strikes older men, many of whom die from something else long before a slow-growing prostate tumor would ever threaten their health. Several recent studies show that, against certain types of prostate cancer, watchful waiting can be as effective as surgery or radiation therapy in terms of survival, at least for the first ten years following diagnosis, without any of the negative side effects of those treatments. After ten years, though, more and more men who follow watchful waiting succumb to metastatic disease.

At its core, watchful waiting is nothing more than a calculated risk. You gamble that you will die of something else—old age, a heart attack, emphysema, the complications of a stroke—before a prostate tumor can grow large enough or spread to other parts of the body and present a mortal danger. Reckoning the odds isn't solely a matter of hunch and gut instinct. Researchers have assembled a body of evidence on which to base decisions (see below). Keep in mind that such odds forecasting isn't limited to watchful waiting. In considering surgery or radiation therapy, a man must also figure his chances of complete cure and weigh them against the very real possibility of recurrence and the unwanted side effects of treatment.

"Deciding what to do about prostate cancer is a tough issue for most men," says the MGH's Dr. Michael Barry. "When you detect it early enough, there aren't any symptoms. You hope that by treating the disease at this stage you can prevent metastatic disease in the future. But you aren't certain *if* metastatic disease will happen even without treatment, nor is treatment a guarantee that cancer won't recur. And for that uncertain benefit, all the side effects that accompany treatment appear today, not years down the road." Watchful waiting, he says, allows men to defer those side effects temporarily or permanently.

Watchful waiting's advantages are these:

• It does not cause impotence, loss of sex drive, incontinence, fatigue, diarrhea, or any other side effects. For some men, this is the deciding factor.

• It does not require a four- or five-day hospital stay and several-week recovery period at home, or daily trips to a medical center for seven or eight weeks.

• It doesn't preclude or interfere with any other treatments. A man on watchful waiting can, at any time, choose to switch to surgery, radiotherapy, or hormone therapy, depending on his preference and his doctor's recommendation.

• It's relatively inexpensive, just the cost of three or four visits to the doctor each year and their associated tests.

The big drawback to watchful waiting is its uncertainty. There's no foolproof way to determine in advance if a tumor will grow imperceptibly and stay confined to the prostate. Small size at diagnosis and low Gleason sum (4 or below) are excellent predictors of this but they don't guarantee it. What's more, there's no way of knowing until it happens if a tumor has spread beyond the prostate. For some men, this not knowing is an unacceptably high price to pay. In reality, though, similar uncertainty exists even with surgery and radiation therapy, where relapses following "successful" treatment aren't uncommon and men sometimes wait for years never really knowing if they are cured or not.

The other thing to keep in mind is that watchful waiting does nothing to hinder the growth of a prostate tumor. Every study of this strategy shows that localized prostate cancer, no matter what its stage or Gleason grade, will *always* progress to metastatic disease. Small tumors with low Gleason grades take the longest to spread, but eventually even they will escape the prostate and threaten a man's health.

Given these two big limitations, why do men choose watchful waiting? Personal reasons, mostly. A few just can't decide which treatment to pick and opt for watchful waiting in the meantime. That's really the wrong use of this strategy. Wait too long and what had been a small, localized tumor may become a somewhat larger tumor no longer contained inside the gland. Some men hope to avoid the side effects of treatment, others believe they will probably die of something else before the tumor can become life-threatening.

Raymond, a fifty-nine-year-old lawyer, explains the former reasoning: "This is happening at the worst possible time for me. A year ago I remarried, to a woman who has completely changed my life. Our time in bed is really important to both of us. I can't imagine not being able to make love together and can't imagine how that would change things for us. The numbers that my doctors were throwing at me about impotence and incontinence after treatment convinced me I'd rather try watchful waiting."

Ed, a seventy-eight-year-old former golf pro, describes the latter point of view: "I don't have a whole lot of years left and those I do have I want to enjoy. Surgery and radiation sounded like they could leave me with some problems I would rather not have. My doctor is pretty sure the cancer I have is small and slow-growing. So I'll take the chance and not do anything about it except go for regular checkups and then hope and pray it doesn't turn into a problem."

The Evidence

As mentioned in Chapter 4, lots of men over age fifty have a spot of malignant prostate cells—a tumor or pretumor. Recent estimates suggest that more than 11 million U.S. males work, love, and play with some cancer in their prostates. The overwhelming majority, around 90 percent, will die without ever suspecting they have this cancer. The malignancy is discovered in the other 10 percent; only three of those ten will die because of it. These numbers testify to the slow-growing nature of most prostate tumors.

With the advent of the PSA test, men are increasingly finding tumors that might otherwise have remained invisible. Most stage A1 and B1 tumors are confined to the gland, making them excellent candidates for curative treatment, i.e., surgery or radiotherapy. The question is, do they pose enough of a threat to health and survival that they require aggressive treatment?

Several recent studies have begun to answer this question. Most of them are from Europe, where watchful waiting is an accepted medical strategy. In Sweden, Dr. Jan-Erik Johansson and his colleagues followed 223 men diagnosed with prostate cancer who did not receive either a radical prostatectomy or radiation therapy. Their average age at the start of the study was seventy-one years. Over the next twelve years, 23 (10 percent) of them died as a direct result of prostate cancer while 148 (66 percent) died of other causes. Dr. Gunnar Aus and his associates found much the same thing. They looked at medical records of 514 Swedish men who died between 1988 and 1990, all of whom had been diagnosed years before with prostate cancer. All started out with watchful waiting and, if any symptoms of advanced prostate cancer appeared, switched to hormone therapy. Of those with stage A1 disease, only a handful died of prostate cancer, and the earliest of these was nineteen years after diagnosis. Those with stage A2 disease had a ten-year disease-specific survival of 79 percent—in other words, of the men who died within ten years of diagnosis, only 21 percent died because of prostate cancer.

At the University of Chicago, Dr. Gerald Chodak and his associates combined the data from six important watchful waiting studies and analyzed them all together. The statistics that lie at the heart of modern medicine are more powerful when they deal with large numbers of cases. Gathering and analyzing data from a number of small studies, a technique known as meta-analysis, improves the statistical power and makes the conclusions drawn from a study more reliable. From this combined data they found that only 13 percent of men with well-differentiated prostate cancer died of their disease within ten years of diagnosis. For those with poorly defined tumors, 77 percent died of prostate cancer within ten years.

Other compelling evidence comes from the Prostate Patient Outcomes Research Team, or P-PORT, now headed by Dr. Barry. This federally funded group of specialists from around the country is comparing the outcomes, or results, from surgery, radiation therapy, and watchful waiting. Outcomes include survival as well as side effects and quality of life. "One thing is very clear," they wrote in the *Journal of the American Medical Association*. "Men aged 75 years and older are not likely to benefit from either radiation therapy or radical prostatectomy when compared to watchful waiting." Keep in mind here that this applies to men with a small, well-differentiated tumor. Those with a larger tumor, or one that contains poorly differentiated tissue, generally need more aggressive treatment since their tumors are more likely to grow and spread beyond the prostate.

The P-PORT researchers picked age seventy-five because men that age, on average, live fewer than ten more years. And the best studies of conservative management show that, for ten years after diagnosis, men with well-differentiated prostate-confined cancer die at the same rate whether they have had surgery or radiation therapy, or have chosen to merely monitor the tumor. And those who pick the latter strategy live without having suffered any of the side effects of the two radical treatments.

Even the strongest supporters of watchful waiting point out its major limitation—it only works for men who won't live more than ten years, either because of old age or another illness. After that, men who choose watchful waiting die of prostate cancer at a higher rate than those who choose aggressive treatment. In the Aus study mentioned earlier, for example, 63 percent of the men who lived at least ten years after first being diagnosed for prostate cancer eventually died of the disease.

The Veterans Administration and the National Cancer Institute have begun an important watchful-waiting study called PIVOT, which stands for Prostate Intervention Versus Observation Trial. The designers hope to devise a clinical trial that randomly assigns men to radical treatment or watchful waiting, though this may be difficult to do in an era when men have definite ideas on how they want their cancer to be handled. Even if a perfectly designed and executed study gets under way tomorrow, it will take ten or fifteen years to reach any definitive conclusions, owing to prostate cancer's slow-growing nature.

Who's a Good Candidate?

At Massachusetts General Hospital, we recommend watchful waiting only to a limited group of men—men over seventy-five or those with severe health problems, who have a well-differentiated tumor embedded well inside the prostate, and whose emotional health would clearly deteriorate if they were unable to have an erection.

Any man can choose not to have treatment for prostate cancer. But that's closer to giving up and letting nature take its course, which may mean an unnecessarily shortened life. Watchful waiting is aimed at giving a man the longest possible life with the least amount of time spent coping with the side effects of treatment. Tumor size and grade, PSA, age, health, and personal preference all enter the equation for calculating who is a good candidate.

From a *medical* perspective, the *best* candidates are men who have a small, well-differentiated tumor and who don't realistically expect to live more than another ten years. Personal preference is harder to quantify. The most frequent reason men cite for choosing this strategy is sex. Several of my younger patients have chosen watchful waiting because they had recently remarried and didn't want anything to interfere with their sex lives. This is a risky ploy because they are often in their fifties or sixties and still have many years to live—and many years for their prostate tumor to inevitably grow and spread. Every urologist knows at least one patient who would rather face death than lose his potency.

Watchful waiting may also serve men with stage C (T3) or D prostate cancer who have no symptoms of metastatic disease—no bone pain and no tumor-related urinary problems. Since the disease differs from man to man, there's no way to predict how soon it will make itself felt. Progression to clinical symptoms can happen in a few months or take several years. Monitoring the cancer and starting hormone therapy at the first sign of symptoms is a perfectly reasonable choice (see Chapter 10).

Some men mistakenly use watchful waiting to buy time before deciding on surgery or radiation therapy. Or they hope a new treatment will appear in the next few years that is more effective and has fewer side effects than those currently available. This is not a wise plan. If your prostate cancer is confined to the gland, and you intend to pick a potentially curative treatment, there's no time like the present. Waiting a month or so won't interfere with your chances for a complete cure. Waiting a year or more definitely could.

Living with Watchful Waiting

As its name implies, watchful waiting requires vigilance, usually in the form of a checkup every four to six months. It is important to stick with this schedule since there's no telling what a tumor might do over the course of a few months. These checkups usually include a digital rectal exam to monitor the tumor. Some physicians encourage their patients to establish a "treatment trigger," often a specific PSA level beyond which they will begin active treatment.

During this period, there are several things you should be on the lookout for, changes that may signal that your tumor has begun spreading:

• A sudden change in your ability to urinate. Sometimes a tumor grows into the urethra and blocks the urine stream.

• An unexplained bone fracture. Falling off a ladder or crashing into a tree while skiing doesn't count. When cancer metastasizes to the bones, it can weaken them so much they break with very little strain or stress.

• A nagging pain in your back or legs. If you have a history of back pain, then yours is probably just a continuation of an old injury or disk disease. But if pain comes out of the blue and lingers, mention this to your physician.

While it sounds simple, living with the equivalent of an unpredictable ticking time bomb inside of you that may, or may not, go off actually takes a fair amount of courage and resolve.

12

Coping with Advanced Disease

(with Dr. Donald S. Kaufman and Dr. William U. Shipley)

Not all men discover their prostate cancer while it's still confined to the gland and thus potentially curable. Since the disease usually grows silently and its warning signs closely resemble the normal changes that accompany aging, at least one-third of men newly diagnosed each year have advanced prostate cancer. That means their tumor has spread into tissue around the gland, to lymph nodes, bones, or other sites. Nor are men with prostate-confined cancer immune from developing advanced disease. Neither radical prostatectomy nor radiation therapy can guarantee permanent eradication of prostate cancer—15 percent or more of men with stage A (T1) or stage B (T2) tumors face advanced prostate cancer even after what appears to be successful treatment.

If tumors always stayed put inside the prostate, this kind of cancer wouldn't be quite as worrisome as it is. Relatively few men die from a gland-confined tumor. The spread of cancer cells to other parts of the body, called metastasis, is what turns prostate cancer into a real killer that takes the lives of more than one hundred American men each day. Why? A tumor inside the prostate must grow quite large before it can threaten a man's life. But even a small metastasis can break bones and interfere with brain function or breathing.

Cancer that spreads beyond its gland of origin does not become a different kind of cancer. When cells from a prostate tumor find their way to the lung, settle down, and grow into a tumor, a man does not suddenly have lung cancer. He has metastatic prostate cancer. This new tumor acts like prostate cancer because all of its cells descended from a prostate cell. In other ways, though, metastatic prostate cancer becomes an entirely different beast from gland-confined prostate cancer. For reasons not yet known, tumor cells grow faster and divide more often once they escape the prostate. They are more aggressive about spreading to other parts of the body. And they become less dependent on hormones like testosterone to "fertilize" their growth. Treating prostate-escaped cancer, then, requires different strategies from dealing with the gland-confined version. Even the goals are different: Therapies devised for prostate-confined cancer aim to *cure* the disease while those for advanced prostate cancer primarily try to buy a man more time. The other main goal is controlling symptoms associated with advanced prostate cancer, pain in particular.

Hormone therapy stands as the cornerstone of treatment for advanced prostate cancer. It holds the disease in check for most men. But it doesn't work permanently— almost all tumors eventually become resistant to it. Unfortunately, few backup treatments exist. Chemotherapy, the predominant weapon against a variety of tumors, has little effect against prostate cancer, whether it is confined to the gland or spread around the body. The toxic agents used in chemotherapy usually target cells that are growing and dividing rapidly. (That's why chemotherapy often makes hair fall out—the drugs damage the fast-growing follicles that anchor hair in place and manufacture new hair.) But metastatic prostate-cancer cells don't always fall into that category and chemotherapy invariably leaves behind a reservoir of untouched cells that continue to grow and spread. "In cancer of the prostate, a response to chemotherapy or second-line hormonal approaches is uncommon and, when it does occur, often short-lived," says Dr. Donald Kaufman, an MGH medical oncologist.

Finding the best treatment for advanced prostate cancer depends on many variables. These include the treatment(s) a man has already tried, how far the cancer has spread, and whether or not any noticeable symptoms have appeared. Personal preference and worries are equally important, since every treatment has its own particular constellation of side effects that can interfere with your life—impotence, loss of interest in sex, fatigue, weight loss, and diarrhea, to name a few.

"Like all of us, men with advanced disease want to live as long as they possibly can," says Dr. Kaufman. "But in choosing a treatment a man might want to consider the *kind* of life, as well as the length of life, it offers. Five years of living with impotence and some gastrointestinal upset might not, for some, be as good as three years of living a relatively normal life."

The following sections describe some of the most common approaches to treating advanced prostate cancer. You'll notice many caveats scattered through the discussion. Despite years of research, we haven't yet found a way to permanently stop this disease. In an age when we expect medical science to have all the answers, this can be frustrating. Worse than that, it often encourages men to explore alternative therapies that have little scientific basis and even less success. Some of these are mentioned in the section on alternative therapy.

Once cancer breaks loose from the prostate gland, it usually heads straight for lymph nodes and then to bones. Metastatic tumors in bony tissue can cause intense, hard-to-treat pain that is often the bane of advanced disease. Because pain control is so important an issue, it gets its own chapter (see Chapter 14).

Hormone Therapy

Hormone therapy acts like a medical Maginot Line against metastatic prostate cancer, a chemical barricade designed to slow the spread of malignant cells throughout the body or to inhibit their growth once established in bone, bladder, lymph node, or other tissue. Ideally it works this way: The cells that make up a prostate gland require male hormones like testosterone and other androgens to grow and divide. Since prostate-cancer cells, even those living in bone or lung tissue, trace their lineage back to normal prostate cells, they too at least initially depend on male hormones to trigger growth and division. Cut off the supply of hormones and you deprive tumor cells of this critical signal. Unfortunately, between 10 and 20 percent of men have a tumor that doesn't depend on hormones for growth, thanks to a genetic mutation in the very early tumor. The rest do respond to lowered hormone levels, though not permanently. Over time, most prostate tumors gradually acquire the ability to grow and divide without a hormone signal.

As described in Chapter 10, hormone therapy can be administered surgically with a one-time operation known as an orchiectomy, orchidectomy, or castration. Or a man can take special drugs. Both approaches drastically reduce the amount of testosterone circulating through the bloodstream. (For a more detailed discussion of the mechanics of hormone therapy, see Chapter 10.)

An orchiectomy removes the testes, the two egg-shaped glands that make both sperm and testosterone. It's a simple, low-risk operation usually requiring no overnight hospital stay. Complete recovery usually follows in two to four days. Within hours of the operation, testosterone levels plummet from the average 600 nanograms per deciliter of blood to below fifty. Relief from symptoms such as bone pain or urinary obstruction can begin almost immediately.

Medical therapy stops testosterone production without removing the testes. The hormone estrogen or drugs known as luteinizing-hormone-releasing hormone agonists (LHRH agonists) stop the pituitary gland from making luteinizing hormone, which the testes need to make testosterone. No LH, no testosterone. Today, most men take LHRH agonists such as leuprolide (Lupron) or goserelin (Zoladex) as a monthly injection. Estrogen is taken as a daily pill. For the first few weeks of LHRH therapy, testosterone production actually *increases* before it drops to orchiectomy levels. To make sure this "flare" doesn't swell tumors or worsen symptoms, most men also take an antiandrogen like flutamide (Eulexin) or bicalutamide (Casodex) to block cells from using any available androgens.

"I usually recommend to my patients that they try an LHRH agonist for a few months. If a tumor responds to the subsequent reduction in testosterone levels, then a man can decide to continue with that form of therapy or switch to an orchiectomy. If it doesn't, then he hasn't been put through the orchiectomy for nothing," says MGH urologist Dr. Alex Althausen.

Orchiectomy and drug therapy appear to be equally effective at halting the spread of advanced prostate cancer. A number of studies show that they have comparable effects on disease progression and survival. They also have the same side effects—impotence, loss of interest in sex, occasional hot flashes similar to those experienced by women going through menopause, and breast enlargement. You should decide which treatment is right for you.

• Orchiectomy requires a morning or afternoon in the hospital and a few days recovery at home, then nothing more. Using LHRH agonists means a monthly trip to the doctor's office for an injection. Estrogen pills must be taken every day.

• Estrogen tablets cost about $400 per year. An orchiectomy costs a one-time fee of $2,000 to $3,000 while an LHRH agonist like leuprolide costs at least $4,000 per year for several (hopefully many) years. Medicare and most private insurers cover the cost of an orchiectomy. Estrogens and LHRH agonists might not be covered if your insurance doesn't include pharmaceutical drugs.

• Taking drugs may be psychologically and emotionally easier than having an orchiectomy. "Even though my doctor explained to me that surgery and drugs would accomplish the same thing, something down deep kept telling me not to have an orchiectomy. It's kind of crazy but I just felt like I would be a different man if I chose that route," says seventy-year-old Richard. But for sixty-six-year-old Paul, "I'm still just as much a man as I was before the operation. I don't like knowing that a doctor had to cut off my testicles, but it's going to give me a few more years with my wife, my daughter, and grandchildren."

In addition, some men see the irreversibility of an orchiectomy as a major disadvantage—the testes can't be reattached in the highly unlikely event that someone discovers a "magic bullet" that eradicates metastatic prostate cancer. LHRH agonists, by comparison, offer more control since stopping the drugs usually causes erections and the sex drive to return.

Combined Hormone Therapy

Some physicians believe that an approach known as combined hormone therapy (CHT) or total androgen ablation is the most effective weapon against metastatic or advanced prostate cancer. This strategy assumes that the androgens produced by the adrenal glands stimulate prostate-cancer cells around the body as effectively as testosterone. The adrenal glands can't be surgically removed without drastic consequences, since these glands also make hormones that control blood pressure and energy metabolism. So drugs called antiandrogens are used to blanket the surface of prostate and prostate-cancer cells, making it nearly impossible for circulating testosterone or other androgens to get inside and trigger further growth and division. Medical studies aren't much help in figuring out if combined hormone therapy is really effective. Some suggest it allows men with advanced prostate cancer to live longer, others don't (see page 200 for a discussion of this issue).

Early vs. Delayed Hormone Therapy

Another unresolved issue is the timing of hormone therapy, whether it is monotherapy (an orchiectomy or LHRH agonist alone) or combination therapy. Until recently, physicians traditionally started a man on hormone therapy at the first sign of advanced disease, usually the appearance of bone pain or "hot spots" on a bone scan. Today, a rising PSA level can detect advanced or recurrent disease years before such symptoms surface. Several studies suggest that beginning hormone therapy at the first sign of a rising PSA can increase both disease-free survival and overall survival, especially for men with "minimal disease." In other words, it may delay the onset of symptoms and lengthen life for men with advanced prostate cancer. Not all the evidence supports this, however. A large clinical trial in Europe shows little benefit for early hormone therapy. And some physicians worry that starting too soon won't leave anything in reserve for when symptoms do appear.

How to Choose

Both combined hormone therapy and early hormone therapy *may* delay the onset of symptoms and *may* prolong your life. Both definitely come with side effects that can radically change your life, such as impotence, loss of sex drive, and lethargy. So in a sense you are gambling an uncertain benefit against a known loss. That's a decision you and your partner have to make, possibly with input from a physician or counselor you trust. If an active sex life is important to you and your physician believes it won't hurt to delay hormone therapy, choose that route. If you want to feel you are doing everything in your power to fight your cancer and sex isn't that important, you would be better served by early hormone therapy. Perhaps one of the smartest things you can do is to talk with some men who have already made this decision. Call a local prostate-cancer support group and explain your problem. Odds are you will be put in touch with several others who have been down that road and whose experiences may help you.

Radiation Therapy

If a tumor appears to have spread into muscle, connective tissue, or organs surrounding the prostate gland—stage C (T3) cancer—but has not progressed to lymph nodes or more distant sites, radiation therapy is an option. Sometimes this local spread is discovered as part of the initial diagnosis, often on the basis of a very high PSA. Sometimes it is detected during a radical prostatectomy with the discovery of "positive margins," tumor cells living at the very edge of the tissue removed during surgery. This means cancer cells still linger in the prostate bed. In either case, irradiating the prostate (or the spot where the prostate used to sit) and the region around it may eradicate a no-longer-confined tumor.

The procedure is almost exactly like that used to treat localized prostate cancer. It usually involves thirty to forty visits to a radiotherapy center spread over six or seven weeks. While the actual radiation takes less than a minute or two, the entire visit generally lasts about an hour once you add in waiting time and preparation. (For a more detailed description, see Chapter 9.) Side effects such as diarrhea and fatigue are generally no more severe than they are for men who have external beam radiation alone.

According to Dr. William Shipley, chief of genitourinary radiation oncology at MGH, men with positive margins who undergo radiation are less likely to have a rising postprostatectomy PSA than are men who don't add radiation to their treatment. This usually means that cancer cells aren't continuing to grow and spread. Follow-ups of men treated at the Massachusetts General Hospital show that following a radical prostatectomy about 50 percent of men with stage C (T3) prostate cancer are free of disease (no rising PSA). Adding adjuvant radiotherapy increases that number to 66 percent. However, researchers have not been able to follow men treated with adjuvant radiotherapy for long enough to see if this additional therapy actually allows them to live longer.

Radiation therapy is also used in other ways against advanced prostate cancer. In some men, the tumor that started the disease grows large enough to block a ureter, the tube connecting the bladder to one kidney. A completely blocked ureter can lead to kidney failure, a potentially life-threatening condition. Radiation can shrink this tumor and reopen the ureter. Small doses of radiation to bones harboring one or more metastases can also prevent fractures at tumor-weakened spots. But this can't be repeated if a tumor returns in the same spot, since further irradiation would kill off the remaining healthy cells in the area. Finally, radiation therapy is an invaluable aid for the small percentage of men with advanced prostate cancer who become suddenly paralyzed by a tumor that compresses the spinal cord. It can rapidly shrink the tumor and relieve pressure on this important bundle of nerves.

Radiation therapy also plays an important role in controlling pain, described in Chapter 14.

Surgery

When cancer spreads beyond the prostate, surgery generally isn't an option. Removing the prostate without also removing the impossible-to-see pockets of tumor cells elsewhere in the body would have as much effect on survival as jailing a single Boston mobster would have on organized crime in Chicago. Urologists rarely recommend a radical prostatectomy for men with stage C (T3) or stage D disease. In fact, they usually go out of their way to make sure that cancer has not spread beyond the prostate before going ahead with surgery. But there are a few exceptions to this no-surgery rule.

• Men with advanced prostate cancer commonly experience urinary blockage, caused by a tumor pressing into the urethra. A transurethral resection of the prostate, or TURP, can reopen this channel and banish the hesitancy, dribbling, inability to urinate, or the need to urinate constantly that accompanies an obstructed urethra. The incisionless TURP requires only a one-night hospital stay and limited recovery time. Using an instrument called a resectoscope inserted into the urethral opening of a man's anesthetized penis, a urologist gently carves away tumor tissue crowding into the urinary tube. It's like removing the pulp from an orange without disturbing the peel. (See Chapter 3 for a more detailed description of this procedure.)

When a man with advanced disease has a TURP, the operation is done only to take care of the urinary symptoms caused by his cancer. A TURP at this stage does little to halt the spread of cancer or improve a man's survival. In physicians' terms, it is done with *palliative* intent (easing symptoms) rather than curative intent.

• When a man chooses radiation therapy to cure prostate-confined cancer and the treatment fails, a "salvage prostatectomy" is sometimes an option. Remember, even though radiation destroys the prostate, the gland's remnants remain in the body. Cancer cells that somehow managed to withstand the high-energy beams can begin forming a new tumor. If that new tumor stays inside the now-defunct prostate, surgically removing the gland may cure the cancer.

This operation is fraught with potential problems. Tissue that has been bombarded by radiation every day for seven weeks changes its shape and texture. That makes it more difficult for a urologist to interpret X rays, transrectal ultrasound exams, and CT scans, all of which offer important information on the new tumor. Equally important, irradiated tissue becomes fragile and difficult to handle. It also heals slowly. And that adds up to a much, much greater risk for incontinence and impotence than is associated with a standard radical prostatectomy. Roughly half the men who have this surgery suffer significant incontinence. Serious injury to the rectal wall that requires a permanent ostomy, or artificial opening, for fecal matter is also a possibility.

"A good candidate for salvage prostatectomy must be highly motivated to do everything possible to totally eradicate his cancer, and that includes living with the side effects," says Dr. Peter Scardino, professor and chairman of urology at Baylor College of Medicine in Houston. Other prerequisites include otherwise excellent health, a life expectancy greater than ten years, no evidence of metastatic or distant disease, and a tumor that would have been originally considered curable by surgery—stage A (T1) or stage B (T2.)

At the 1994 meeting of the American College of Surgeons, Dr. Scardino reported on the Baylor team's experience with this procedure, involving forty men over eight years. Thirty-five were still alive, two had died of recurrent prostate cancer, and two had died of other causes. One man could not be located for follow-up. Some of the thirty-five survivors had a rising PSA, but no symptoms of advanced disease.

This operation clearly isn't for everyone. The men in the Baylor series aren't representative of the average man with radiation-treated prostate cancer. The researchers carefully selected only those men they thought could withstand the operation. Furthermore, they have not been able to collect information about long-term survival and disease progression. Due to the slow-growing nature of prostate cancer we won't know for another few years if this is really a viable operation in terms of added survival.

• At the Mayo Clinic in Rochester, Minnesota, Dr. Horst Zincke and his associates have been removing cancerous prostate glands from men in whom the disease has spread to lymph nodes or other more distant sites (stage D). Doing this, they reason, decreases the body's tumor burden. Removing the cancer's home base could mean fewer cells available to colonize other parts of the body. These men are also started on hormone therapy just before surgery, making it impossible to determine if any advantage is from the prostatectomy or the hormone therapy. Few other urologists have adopted this technique.

Cryosurgery

Some men turn to cryosurgery when cancer persists in the prostate gland after radiation therapy. It is *not* an option when tumor cells have spread to lymph nodes, the bladder, bones, or other tissues.

This technique freezes the prostate using a supercold mixture of liquid nitrogen. The frozen tissue dies just as skin tissue does after prolonged frostbite. (See page 157 for a detailed description of the process.) Since no incisions are required, recovery is generally faster than with traditional open surgery. In fact, recovery after cryosurgery is closer to recovery after a TURP—one day in the hospital and about a week at home.

While cryosurgery appears to be what researchers euphemistically call a "promising" technique for treating persistent cancer in an irradiated prostate, there really aren't reliable data on which to base this kind of judgment. The first modern cryosurgeries were performed in 1990, and five years of follow-up just isn't enough time to tell if it will be effective at eradicating or controlling persistent, gland-confined tumors. Researchers at a handful of institutions where this procedure has been used for several years report high negative biopsy rates at six months and one year, but none has been able to evaluate whether this procedure prevents prostate cancer from spreading to other tissues or adds months or years to a man's life.

What cryosurgeons have discovered is that the technique isn't free of side effects, especially in men who have had prior radiation or a TURP. At Allegheny General Hospital in Pittsburgh, where modern prostate cryosurgery got its start in 1990, substantial incontinence afflicts somewhere between 10 and 30 percent of men who opt for this treatment when cancer persists following radiation therapy, says Dr. Ralph Miller, an assistant professor of surgery at the Medical College of Pennsylvania and an Allegheny cryosurgeon. Rates of significant stress incontinence reach much higher. Cryosurgery also leads to impotence at least 50 percent of the time it is used for persistent prostate cancer. On top of the 50 percent of men already impotent after radiation therapy, few men have erections following this double-barreled approach. There's an even more devastating side effect that occurs in one to two men per 100 who have cryosurgery. The wall of the rectum, which sits only a few millimeters away from the prostate, sometimes freezes during the procedure. This opens a permanent hole that can't always be surgically repaired. A man with an irreparable fistula must excrete solid waste through an ostomy, or permanent opening on his abdomen.

Given what we know right now, cryosurgery for prostate-confined cancer that persists following radiation therapy is a gamble. It is associated with decent negative biopsy rates and low PSA levels, suggesting that it has either halted or eradicated the cancer. But there are no data showing that men who have adjuvant cryosurgery live any longer than men who don't. And there's plenty of data showing that they suffer side effects at a fairly high rate.

When Hormone Therapy Fails

About 20 percent of men with prostate cancer don't respond to hormone therapy at all. Their tumors continue to grow even when testosterone and androgen levels are at rock bottom. And while the majority of men *do* respond to hormone therapy, the benefits don't last indefinitely. At some point, tumor cells either adapt to low hormone levels or hormone-independent clusters of cells come to dominate tumors.

In either case, almost every man with advanced prostate cancer will eventually need something besides standard hormone therapy to battle his disease. This is where treatment decisions get murky. Hormone-insensitive or hormone-resistant prostate cancer is extraordinarily difficult to stop. Standard chemotherapy agents that have been so successful against other kinds of cancer usually have little effect against this one. None tried so far offers predictable pain relief or increases survival. At best, only 20 to 30 percent of men who try such second-line treatments benefit from them. Does that mean you shouldn't try one of the many options that are under investigation? *No!* Remember, while the average response may not be good, some men do beautifully. But keep in mind that the side effects may be quite unpleasant.

Most advanced therapies are still classified as experimental and thus aren't available in every hospital or medical center. You may have to enroll in a clinical study at a nearby cancer center or travel to a distant city. Some of the more promising therapies are listed in figure 12.1 (page 237). You can get an updated list that includes the name and phone number of the study director by calling the national Cancer Information Service at 800-4-CANCER and asking for a list of current clinical trials or protocols for advanced prostate cancer. Or if your public library has access to the National Cancer Institute/National Library of Medicine's PDQ data base, you can get the same information from it.

Advanced treatments fall into four main categories—secondary hormone therapy, cell-killing chemotherapy, growth-factor inhibitors, and vaccines and antibodies.

Secondary Hormone Therapy

When hormone monotherapy can no longer keep advanced prostate cancer in check, adding daily doses of an antiandrogen like flutamide (Eulexin) or bicalutamide (Casodex) is a common next step. This so-called total androgen blockade prevents cells from absorbing any androgens that still remain in circulation. Depriving prostate-cancer cells of these hormones may stunt their growth or stop it altogether. Some men whose cancers are progressing despite an orchiectomy or LHRH therapy respond to antiandrogen therapy. Others don't, possibly because their tumors no longer depend on hormone stimulation.

Another second-line hormone approach uses prednisone, a glucocorticoid hormone commonly used to control asthma, to stop inflammation from poison ivy, or to alleviate arthritis pain. It decreases the levels of two hormones, dehydroepiandrosterone and androsteindione, which may stimulate prostate-cancer-cell growth.

Several drug therapies shut off androgen production inside the adrenal glands. A drug called ketoconazole (Nizoral), originally developed to kill fungal infections, corrupts certain enzymes in the adrenal glands and prevents them from turning cholesterol and other complex compounds into steroid hormones, including androgens. This drug may also kill tumor cells. In clinical trials, up to 30 percent of men derive some benefit from ketoconazole—less pain or reduction in urinary obstruction—though it does not appear to lengthen life. Because ketoconazole works so quickly, it is most often suggested for men who have symptoms that appear suddenly and demand immediate resolution. The downside of this drug is that it can damage the liver, produce intense nausea and vomiting, and lead to anorexia, which further weakens a man already sapped by prostate cancer and therapy. The side effects usually limit the use of ketoconazole to a few weeks; its long-term effects are being investigated.

Aminoglutethimide (Cytadren) is another drug that squelches androgen production. It too can sometimes alleviate the symptoms associated with advanced prostate cancer. Men taking this drug must also take daily doses of a steroid hormone like hydrocortisone to replace critical hormones for energy metabolism that are turned off as well. Skin rashes, thyroid problems, and fatigue often accompany this treatment.

Chemotherapy

Circulating a toxic drug throughout the body kills cells. Since drugs can't discriminate between good and bad, they kill tumor cells, follicle cells, skin cells, cells lining the stomach and intestine, and other fast-growing cells. Side effects of chemotherapy such as hair loss, skin rashes, nausea, and vomiting attest to the fact that these drugs work. So does the survival of millions of people who beat Hodgkin's disease, testicular cancer, or leukemia. Unfortunately, no chemotherapy agents tested so far halt the spread of metastatic prostate cancer or routinely send the disease into remission. Perhaps some of the research efforts currently under way may change that in the future. Why bother trying chemotherapy, then? There's always hope that a new drug, or new combination of old drugs, could make a difference. And some of these drugs do help relieve pain when painkillers don't.

A long list of compounds have been turned against hormone-insensitive prostate cancer, alone and in various combinations. These include doxorubicin, cisplatin, methotrexate, 5-fluorouracil, cyclophosphamide, estramustine, and mitomycin-C. A list of those under investigation by National Cancer Institute–affiliated researchers is listed in figure 12.1. Other compounds are being used or studied in less formal ways all over the country. A call to PAACT or Us-Too, a posting on the Internet, or a computer bulletin board can probably turn up some of these efforts.

You take some of these drugs in pill form. Others require a daily trip to a physician's office or medical center for intravenous administration. A few even require that you be fitted with a small, portable pump that constantly infuses the drug or drug combination into your bloodstream all day long as you work, meet friends, or rest.

Since chemotherapy is still considered experimental treatment for advanced prostate cancer, many insurers will not pay for it. Medicare, for example, generally doesn't pay for any infusion therapy for prostate cancer. Since al-

Figure 12.1. Drugs that may fight prostate cancer currently being investigated by the National Cancer Institute

5-fluorouracil	lovastatin
allopurinol	mitomycin-C
aminoglutethimide	mitoxantrone
carboplatin	paclitaxel (Taxol)
cimetidine	phenylacetate
cyclophosphamide	phenylbutyrate
cyproterone acetate	shark cartilage
docetaxel (Taxotere)	suramin
doxorubicin	tamoxifen
estramustine	topotecan
etoposide	vinblastine
isoretinoin	

most all these drugs are quite costly, your best bet is to enroll in an approved clinical study where the drugs are provided free of charge.

Growth-Factor Inhibitors

Testosterone and androgens aren't the only substances that stimulate normal and cancerous cells. Our bodies produce an army of small proteins called growth factors that trigger cell growth and division. Suppressing their production or activity, or blocking cells from recognizing them, could theoretically halt the growth and spread of metastatic prostate tumors. So could preventing new blood vessels from growing toward the tumor and connecting it to nutrients in the circulatory system. Early results suggest that this theory is still way ahead of the practice. But given all the ongoing research, there's hope this approach will eventually pay off against prostate and other cancers.

Using growth-factor inhibitors against tumors is a field in its infancy, so few proven successes have been reported. A drug called suramin, which was originally developed to kill a blood-cell parasite, has generated some excitement among prostate-cancer researchers. Suramin binds to a number of growth factors and essentially disguises them. Cells can't recognize the suramin–growth-factor complex and thus can't absorb the critical growth factor. In two small clinical trials, suramin reduced PSA levels in half the men taking the drug. (Lower PSA readings indicate the drug either slowed the growth of existing tumor cells or killed some.) About 70 percent of the men reported less pain while taking suramin. Unfortunately, the drug's side effects sometimes outweighed its potential benefits—a substantial number of men stop taking the drug because of kidney problems, nausea and vomiting, and circulatory problems.

Immunotherapy

For more than a decade, researchers have been searching for ways to make the body's own immune system fight cancer. Despite intriguing experiments and countless person-hours of laboratory work, this approach is still highly experimental and doesn't yet offer a cancer cure, or even reliable relief from cancer pain. Still, the ongoing work appears to be moving toward those goals, though at a snail's pace.

One approach relies on what have been dubbed "magic bullets" against cancer. This radical form of therapy uses small molecules called monoclonal antibodies to seek out and kill tumor cells no matter where they are in the body or how few might be in any one place. Monoclonal-antibody therapy begins with tumor cells removed from a man's cancerous prostate. These are injected into a mouse or rabbit. The animal makes natural antibodies against proteins on the foreign cells' surfaces. The antibodymaking cells are then removed from the animal's spleen and grown in culture to produce as many antitumor antibodies as possible. They are called monoclonal antibodies because they come from one kind of rabbit or mouse cell. Once enough have been manufactured, they are injected into the man from whom the prostate tumor cells were initially removed. In theory, the monoclonal antibodies latch on to proteins found only on cancer cells in his system and make adjacent cells clump together. Cells in the body's immune system recognize and attack these clumps more readily than they go after unclumped cancer cells.

Some researchers are taking this approach a step further and attaching cell-killing drugs to the monoclonal antibodies. They would act as special delivery agents, bringing radioactive or toxic compounds directly to tumor cells and avoiding healthy cells. The most promising of these so far is called tumor-necrosis treatment. The active agent in this is a monoclonal antibody made to recognize a protein called tumor-necrosis factor (TNF) that is produced by cancer cells, especially those that are old or dying. In theory, anti-TNF monoclonal antibodies will home in on tumors and make them more recognizable to white blood cells, the body's scavengers.

Alternative Therapy

Physicians, naturopathic healers, nutrition experts, gurus, and a host of others offer dozens of alternatives to the medical therapies described above. They range from macrobiotic diets and coffee enemas to injections of shark cartilage, breathing the highly reactive form of oxygen known as ozone, taking potions of plant extracts or supposedly curative chemicals, and spiritual exercises designed to bring harmony to an "unbalanced" body and purge the cancer. In *A Private Battle,* a very personal memoir about his ultimately unsuccessful fight against prostate cancer, Cornelius Ryan describes one example of an alternative therapy. Someone suggested that he eat an Eskimo soup "made from the bloods of animals and mixed with the stomach and intestinal contents as well." The author of *The Longest Day* declined the opportunity.

Do any nontraditional therapies work? That's extremely hard to say. Virtually every alternative healer can tell you about two or three individuals, perhaps more, whose cancer disappeared when they started following his or her advice. But many of these people were simultaneously undergoing conventional medical therapy. In the widely read book *Recalled by Life*, Dr. Anthony Sattilaro chronicled his diagnosis in July 1978 with advanced prostate cancer and his discovery of a macrobiotic diet— eating primarily cooked vegetables and whole grains while avoiding sugar and processed foods. He ends the book in August 1981 after a negative bone scan with these words: "I was diagnosed by my physicians as in complete remission." At the same time, however, Dr. Sattilaro had undergone an orchiectomy, which can also make cancer disappear. However, the remission wasn't permanent, and the author died ten years later of recurrent prostate cancer.

So far, no alternative therapy has ever been tested as rigorously as the more traditional ones commonly used to fight early or advanced prostate cancer. This means treating a large group of men with similar-stage tumors, half with no therapy or standard therapy and half with the alternative, then watching how long it takes for the disease to progress and how long the men live. Such head-to-head comparisons just don't exist.

A surprisingly large number of men with advanced prostate cancer turn to alternative therapies. That's not surprising, since medical approaches offer little hope once hormone therapy stops working. Alternative treatments offer that hope plus an unmeasurable something else—the feeling that you are taking control of your health and your treatment. That emotional shift may improve your attitude and sense of how you are feeling. Even if it adds little in the way of extra survival, that may be an important benefit. But before you abandon the traditional route and opt for something less mainstream, take a long, skeptical look at the options that others peddle.

• Effectiveness aside, many alternative therapies are harmless. They won't hurt you, even though they may not help. A few, on the other hand, can be hazardous to your health. Repeated coffee enemas, which some practitioners believe increase the body's ability to rid itself of toxic products, can cause serious fluid imbalances. One alternative therapy that included raw calf-liver juice contaminated cancer patients with bacteria that caused serious intestinal infections and several deaths. So ask a physician you trust to evaluate a potentially attractive alternative therapy, at least for its ability to do you harm.

• You end up making a decision about advanced therapies at a time when you are particularly vulnerable. Other treatments aren't working, and you want so badly to stay healthy and alive. Sometimes hope pushes logic and critical thinking aside. You really need to view each new, promising opportunity with a huge dose of skepticism. If someone you didn't know were to call you on the telephone and ask you to invest several thousand dollars in a "surefire opportunity," odds are you'd hang up, or at least check out the scheme with a reputable investor. Your life is worth more than a few thousand dollars, so do the same with an alternative treatment. Ask tough questions and demand some facts. Is the therapy specifically for prostate cancer or is it a general anticancer therapy? Has it been tested in real clinical trials or are there just testimonials from those who believe in its power? How many men have tried it? How old were they and what stage tumors did they have? How many of those men are alive five and ten years later?

• The other thing you might want to consider is cost. With the exception of a macrobiotic diet, which you can do yourself, alternative therapies aren't free or even inexpensive. They can run into the tens of thousands of dollars—few of which Medicare or a private insurer will cover. Make sure you get up front an idea of the overall cost.

A few of the more common alternative therapies are briefly described below. (*Choices in Healing*, a new book by Michael Lerner, covers a host of alternative therapies in great but not overwhelming detail.) Despite the often-glowing reports from alternative practitioners, none of these techniques has been proven effective in careful clinical trials.

Laetrile

The trade name for a substance related to amygdalin, a compound extracted from the pits of apricots and other fruits. It is sometimes erroneously called vitamin B17. Laetrile was first used to treat cancer patients in the 1950s, and enjoyed some popularity in the 1960s and 1970s. Despite reports that laetrile was responsible for cancer cures, or at least for holding the disease at bay, a rigorous scientific test showed the treatment offered little value. Researchers at the Mayo Clinic tested the compound against a variety of advanced tumors for which there was no cure at the time. Of 175 patients they could evaluate, only one showed a "partial response" and that disappeared after a short time. In fact, by the end of the three-week treatment period, more than half of those enrolled in the study showed clear signs of disease progression, and 80 percent showed continuing disease after two months. In reporting their results, the researchers concluded in the *New England Journal of Medicine* that survival times were "consistent with the anticipated survivals in comparable patients receiving inactive or no treatment" at all.

GERSON THERAPY

Cancer occurs when the body loses its resistance to disease and its ability to heal itself because of "artificial nutrition," according to Dr. Max Gerson. Beginning in the 1930s, he promoted a cancer treatment aimed at restoring both of these. The two main elements were a diet that included only fresh fruits and vegetables supplemented with fresh calf-liver juice, vitamins, and other extracts and included regular coffee enemas to remove toxins from the system. Although Dr. Gerson died in 1959, a number of clinics in the United States, Mexico, and elsewhere still offer this therapy or a variation on it.

ANTINEOPLASTONS

Stanislaw Burzynski, M.D., has spent his life isolating and researching a series of small protein fragments from human urine. He believes that these fragments, dubbed antineoplastons, form a crucial part of the body's natural defense system against "the enemy from within"—errors in cell programming that may lead to cancer or other diseases. Operating out of his own clinic and research institute in Houston, Texas, Dr. Burzynski has tested antineoplastons (combined with DES, an estrogen hormone often used as part of standard hormone therapy) in what appear to be standard clinical trials against advanced, hormone-resistant prostate cancer. The results were promising enough that researchers affiliated with traditional medical schools have begun their own tests, and the new federal Office of Alternative Medicine has approved an antineoplaston clinical trial.

SHARK CARTILAGE

Since this therapy was given some rather uncritical national exposure on the television program *60 Minutes*, its stock has soared among alternative practitioners. Four substances in shark cartilage appear to prevent the growth of new blood vessels, an activity that cancer cells must orchestrate in order to survive. Without new blood vessels, a tumor can't get dissolved food from the bloodstream or dispose of cellular wastes. In his 1993 book *Sharks Don't Get Cancer,* author William Lane exaggerated the promise of shark cartilage. For one, sharks *do* get cancer, something he now admits. For another, the active substances in shark cartilage—and cow cartilage, for that matter—have been under investigation since the 1970s. While such antiangiogenesis factors appear promising, they haven't yet been shown to cure cancer or stop its spread.

Shark cartilage isn't difficult to get. The FDA calls it a nontoxic substance, so dozens of companies now make shark cartilage capsules and sell them through the mail or in virtually any natural-food or natural-health store. Before you pick up a bottle and begin a do-it-yourself cancer therapy, check with your physician to make sure that it won't make an existing heart or other condition worse. If you'd rather try shark cartilage and contribute to our knowledge about this substance, see if you can enroll in one of the ongoing clinical trials. You can get information from the National Cancer Institute or call the National Institutes of Health's newly established Office of Alternative Medicine. (See Resources.)

ESSIAC

Beginning in the 1920s, a Canadian nurse named Rene Caisse treated her cancer patients with an infusion made from four plants—sheep sorrel, slippery elm, Turkish rhubarb, and burdock root—that she learned from a Native American medicine man. This herbal mixture supposedly cured many people suffering with terminal cancer. Available today as Essiac (that's Caisse spelled backward) it appears to have some medicinal properties. In fact, a small trial that Caisse and researchers from Northwestern University conducted in the late 1930s showed that her infusion may have prolonged life and diminished pain in people with terminal cancer. One warning—the mixture contains high levels of oxalic acid, which could make it dangerous for people with arthritis or those with kidney problems.

VISUALIZATION

The imagination has become an increasingly important tool for both alternative and mainstream practitioners. What's called creative visualization is being used to help people withstand the stress of having cancer and being treated for it. Some proponents go further and claim that visualization may actually help halt or even destroy cancer. Perhaps the best-known proponents of this technique are the team of O. Carl Simonton, M.D., and Stephanie Matthews Simonton, who operate a clinic in Houston, Texas. Their book *Getting Well Again* makes the case for visualization and offers simple, do-it-yourself steps. Basically the Simontons and others recommend that you first use meditation or a progressive relaxation technique to focus on the task ahead. Once you are relaxed and focused, you try to picture cancer cells as weak, confused, easily destroyed cells. At the same time you conjure up an image of your own cells—especially your white blood cells—as strong, healthy, and ready for battle. Then you follow the image to its logical conclusion, perhaps taking great satisfaction with the way your healthy cells search out and destroy the cancerous ones.

Does visualization work? That's hard to say. On the *medical* level, the evidence is slim to nonexistent that visualization alone works as well as or better than traditional cancer therapies. Combining this technique with traditional therapy, however, may increase the latter's effectiveness. On a *personal* level, visualization may definitely help, since it makes the visualizer a more active participant in his therapy. And it appears to have no harmful side effects.

Nutrition

As mentioned in Chapter 5, there's evidence that diet and prostate cancer are somehow linked. A 1994 study from Harvard Medical School, for example, suggests that a high-fat diet may rev up tiny, slow-growing, and otherwise indolent tumors. The study, which followed the health and diet of more than 50,000 physicians from 1986 to 1990, found that men who ate meal-sized portions of red meat five or more times a week were more likely to develop advanced prostate cancer than those who ate red meat less than once a week.

If poor nutrition might *cause* prostate cancer, can good nutrition slow its progress? Researchers from Tulane University School of Public Health asked that very question and did a small study to get an answer. They compared eighteen men with stage D2 disease, all of whom were following standard hormone therapy. Half of the men ate a high-fiber, low-fat diet, the others their normal diet. The men in the high-fiber group lived an average of 228 months, compared to seventy-eight months for the control group. While the results are intriguing, the study was so small that they may have been due to chance alone—if other researchers were to repeat this work they might find just the opposite. Further study is undoubtedly needed.

Even without such a study, though, good nutrition can clearly make a difference in your fight against prostate cancer. The healthier and better fortified you are, the more you'll be able to tolerate treatment and avoid side effects. Eating well also keeps your already overburdened immune system in shape. Not only is it doing its "normal" job of recognizing and destroying foreign invaders like bacteria and viruses, it's working overtime trying to battle the invaders from within.

No one yet knows how or why, but many kinds of tumors speed up the body's metabolism while at the same time depressing appetite. The result is a progressive weight loss that physicians call cancer cachexia. This cachexia, or wasting, can become so severe that it actually causes death, rather than the tumor itself. The best way to protect yourself from cancer-related malnutrition is to eat as well as you possibly can. Try to eat three real meals a day, and don't be afraid to snack in between. High-calorie supplements are an option, but real food with its full complement of vitamins, minerals, and trace elements is probably much better. Your physician may recommend special drinks, or even intravenous feeding at night, to help keep your weight up.

13

Coping with Incontinence and Impotence

It's a cruel twist of fate that the prostate isn't as cancer-free as other important organs like the heart or spleen. Cruel because this golf-ball-sized orb of tissue sits strategically at the intersection of two crucial functions—urination and sex. As a result, symptoms of the disease or side effects of treatment often disrupt urinary or sexual function. To make matters worse, most men find it difficult to talk about either of these two normal, natural activities. Privacy, modesty, and embarrassment prevent some men from telling their physicians about these problems. Others try desperately to hide them from partners, children, friends, and colleagues.

Prostate cancer interferes with urinary and sexual function in a variety of ways. An untreated or advanced tumor can invade and weaken one of several muscles needed to control urine flow. Or a large tumor can bulge into the urethra and block the urine stream. Ironically, incontinence and impotence are even more likely to arise as side effects of the two main treatments for prostate cancer, surgery and radiation therapy. Both of these can cause intermittent or complete urinary incontinence. And both can destroy the ability to have an erection. Hormone therapy, in addition to interfering with erections, also quenches the desire for sex.

Before treatment, men worry more about impotence than incontinence. Afterward, however, the reality of incontinence usually proves to be the more devastating issue. Even the most sexually active man urinates many more times each week than he has sex. And urination can't be postponed until bedtime or the weekend. The urge arises constantly throughout the day, often in the middle of a job, a dinner, a hand of cards. And it's a far more public function. One man put it this way: "The guy sitting next to you on the subway won't ever have a clue if you are impotent or not. But he sure might know you are incontinent if you've suddenly sprung a leak or have a saturated pad that smells."

This isn't to downplay the sense of loss and frustration that accompanies treatment-related impotence. "Losing the ability to have an erection is a striking blow to many men, even to those who stopped having sex years before," says Patricia Perri Rieker, director of psychosocial research at the Dana Farber Cancer Institute in Boston, who has been studying how men respond to prostate cancer for years. "Deep down, many men equate erections with maleness. Losing that ability, then, can mean the loss of manhood. And it's compounded by the fact that this disease often appears right around retirement, when a man is also giving up the work by which he defined himself for many years."

Incontinence and impotence aren't necessarily permanent. Though most men are incontinent immediately after prostate surgery, urine control can be restored as nerves and tissues heal, swelling subsides, and strength and muscle tone return. Erectile function can take longer to reappear and isn't as resilient as continence.

This chapter explains how prostate cancer and its treatments can cause impotence and incontinence, and how you can master these setbacks, or at least adapt to them. Each section starts with a quick tour of the relevant anatomy, then concentrates on coping strategies that range from exercises and changes in behavior to medical and surgical fixes.

Incontinence

Anatomy

The prostate sits directly below the bladder, held to it by a band of connective tissue. Tough, fibrous tissue also anchors the prostate to the nearby pubic bone and firmly holds it in the pelvic cavity. The gland surrounds, and becomes part of, the tube that carries urine from bladder to penis. Like an apple core and pulp, it's impossible to tell where the urethra ends and the prostate begins. The bladder, a crucial player in continence and incontinence, is basically an expandable balloon for holding fluid surrounded by a muscular coat. Urine enters the bladder from the kidneys via a right and left ureter; it exits via the urethra.

Four separate sets of muscles normally control a man's urine flow. Muscles around the bladder (1) initiate urination by contracting. This squeezes the bladder and forces urine toward the only outlet. Where bladder meets prostate, the bladder-neck muscles (2) act as the first "dam" against urine flow. Muscles inside the prostate (3) automatically keep the gland wrapped around the urethra, generating substantial resistance against urine flow. And the pelvic floor muscles (4), technically called the pubococcygeal muscles, provide a second dam against urine. This final barrier, called the external sphincter, is the same muscle that surrounds the anus. It's the one you tighten to prevent passing gas or to control a bowel movement. All of these muscle groups are under automatic or unconscious control, otherwise you'd never stay dry at night. But they can be consciously overridden—before embarking on a long car trip, for example, you can make yourself urinate before getting a full-bladder signal.

As the bladder fills near its capacity, a sensor signals the brain that it's high time for an emptying. This registers physically as well, with a feeling of fullness in the lower abdomen and a characteristic sensation in the penis. A man without prostate problems can resist this signal for quite some time before the need to urinate becomes urgent. Once he acknowledges it's time to go, he finds the closest bathroom, men's room, or private tree on the golf course, unzips his pants and then, after a second or two, starts urinating. This seemingly simple function actually requires extraordinary coordination. Not until everything is ready—man standing at urinal, pants unzipped, penis pointing at the white basin—does the brain signal the bladder-neck, prostate, and pelvic-floor muscles to relax. This opens the floodgates, and the contracting bladder propels urine through the urethra and out the tip of the penis. As the bladder finishes emptying, the bladder-neck muscles tighten and choke off the outflow. Conscious contractions of the external sphincter expel any urine remaining in the urethra; then it, too, clamps the tube shut.

Types of Incontinence

The term "incontinence" is really a catch phrase for several distinct problems. These problems can arise for a host of reasons such as muscle degeneration, bladder irritability, or side effects from common drugs—they are not solely linked with prostate cancer. In fact, men with prostate-cancer-related urinary problems are a minority of men with incontinence.

Four types of urine-control problems commonly occur in men with prostate cancer, or following treatment for it:

STRESS INCONTINENCE

A faulty washer in the urethral faucet causes a squirt or two of urine to gush out of the penis whenever pressure is put on the bladder. This is called stress incontinence. It can accompany coughing, sneezing, a belly laugh, bending or sitting down, lifting a heavy object, climbing stairs, or throwing a bowling ball. All of these tighten the abdomen and compress the bladder. Normally, the body automatically compensates for these sudden, instantaneous changes by further tightening sphincter or bladder-neck muscles and thus raising the dam against urine flow even higher than normal. A damaged or missing bladder neck or a weak external sphincter can't contract hard enough or fast enough to counter these pressure changes.

URGE INCONTINENCE

A misbehaving bladder leads to urge incontinence. For men with this condition powerful, undeniable urges to urinate come out of the blue. They rarely give a man time to hurry to the nearest bathroom, and can cause rather large accidents. A bladder made irritable or unstable by radiation contracts unpredictably, often without first alerting the other players in the urinary reflex. Benign prostatic hyperplasia (BPH) can also cause an irritable bladder.

Overflow Incontinence

The kidneys continually send urine to the bladder, gradually expanding it until the "empty" signal is triggered. If something blocks the only outlet, the urethra, or if damaged bladder muscles can no longer contract as they should, the bladder won't empty normally. When this happens, the overflow leaks into the urethra and constantly dribbles out the penis. This often happens to men with BPH, when the enlarged prostate compresses the urethra like a clamp around a radiator hose. Scar tissue growing after radiation treatment or prostate surgery can also jut into the urethral canal and impede urine flow, leading to overflow incontinence.

Urinary Obstruction

Sometimes a tumor or stricture can completely block the urethra, making urination impossible. The resulting over-full bladder hurts and must be drained promptly in a doctor's office or hospital emergency room. If it is not, the kidneys back up and stop working, a critical situation that can be deadly. Obstruction can occur gradually, but it can also appear without warning. You might notice a sudden change in voiding, like being able to squeeze out only a few drops.

Draining an obstructed bladder is a relatively simple

procedure. A hollow, flexible tube called a catheter is inserted into the penis, through the urethra, and into the bladder. Backed-up urine drains out, offering immediate relief. If acute urinary retention is caused by something blocking the urethra, the catheter may have to be pushed through the abdomen directly into the bladder.

How Treatment Causes Problems

By definition, a radical prostatectomy generally eliminates two levels of control—the bladder-neck muscles and the prostate itself. The former are often unavoidably severed or damaged during the operation, and the latter is always removed. Most men overcome these losses and retrain their bodies with special sphincter-strengthening exercises that return urinary control. Others wear an absorbent pad in their shorts to catch the occasional dribble of urine. But damage the external sphincter and persistent trouble arises. In order to achieve clean margins, a surgeon must sometimes take a fair amount of tissue from around the prostate gland. This swath may involve the external sphincter. Or the inevitable tugging, pulling, and slicing that occurs during the course of an operation may harm these muscles. This leaves a man with no effective mechanisms to control urine flow and often results in complete incontinence. Radiation therapy damages the external sphincter far less often, though it does happen. More likely, irradiation irritates the bladder and causes persistent urge incontinence.

At Massachusetts General Hospital and other medical centers where expert surgeons routinely perform prostatectomies, less than 1 percent of men develop severe incontinence. Following radiation therapy only about 1 to 2 percent of men develop severe incontinence. At other centers where these procedures aren't done as often, the rates are much higher. A survey of 200 Boston-area men one year after treatment for early stage prostate cancer may give a more representative tally of incontinence rates. Of those who had chosen to have a radical prostatectomy, 40 percent reported regularly wearing pads in their underwear during the previous four weeks and 13 percent reported leaking urine "a lot." The numbers for postirradiation incontinence were 5 percent and 2 percent.

The vast majority of men are incontinent immediately after a radical prostatectomy, at least for a few weeks. When the Foley catheter comes out, the weakened and traumatized urinary system just isn't up to controlling the flow. Some kind of pad or adult diaper (see below) must be used. It takes time for any swelling to subside, for internal healing to occur, and for nerves and muscles to recover from being cut and pushed around. Depending on how fast you heal, continence should begin returning in two to six months. The first sign you'll probably notice is waking up dry some morning. Next comes improved continence early in the day, before you and your urinary system tire out. Late afternoon and evening continence are usually the last to return—in some men it takes months. Full recovery, or as full as you will get, may take from twelve to twenty-four months. The exercises described below can be invaluable in speeding return.

"At the very least, a man should wait three to four months before getting worried about permanent incontinence after a radical prostatectomy. After that, he should definitely see his urologist or primary-care physician for a good physical workup and possibly some specialized tests," says MGH urologist Dr. Alex Althausen.

Taking Action

Incontinence is a frustrating, potentially embarrassing problem. It can make one avoid friends or change habits. One man retired earlier than he had planned. Another stopped going to church or social functions. One man stopped flying from Boston to Seattle to visit his daughter and grandchildren. Another stopped having sex because he couldn't hold his urine during intimate moments.

Fortunately, most men don't have to make such big changes or sacrifices. Thanks to a variety of exercises and devices, most men can limit or even reverse incontinence. If you are having trouble keeping dry, admit to yourself you're having a problem. Then do something about it. First off, talk to someone who can help. Call your urologist and arrange an appointment specifically to talk about bladder control. If past experience tells you that he or she won't take the time you need to talk and explore different options, get a referral from your primary-care physician for another specialist. Or call a large hospital or medical center in your area; many have special incontinence clinics. Other good resources are Help for Incontinent People, a national support and information group, and members of a local prostate cancer support network. (See Resources for addresses and telephone numbers.) Through each of these you can find caring incontinence experts in your area.

Before meeting with an incontinence specialist, try what Mario, a seventy-four-year-old barber, did for two weeks when his postprostatectomy incontinence didn't seem to be getting any better. "I kept track of every time I had to urinate, when and how much I drank, and what I was doing at the time. When I brought it to my doctor, he could see right away I had mostly stress incontinence," he says. Experts recommend keeping such a bladder diary. Make a note every time you urinate or lose urine. Include the time, the amount, and what prompted it—a cough, a sudden urge, lifting something at work, etc. Write down what you drink and when. Also record any over-the-counter medications you're taking—some can interfere with urine control. Such a record can prove invaluable in revealing the difference between urge and stress incontinence, or pointing out possible changes in your daily routine that may make a difference. It also makes you more involved in your own care and therapy.

A range of options exist for men with incontinence. A pad, clamp, or catheter can keep a man's clothes dry, but none of these minimizes or corrects the problem. At-home exercises cost nothing but offer an excellent chance for regaining control. If those aren't enough, drugs, injections, or a surgically implanted artificial sphincter may be needed. The nature of your problem, your own physiology and health, your determination and desire all affect how long it will take for you to conquer incontinence. For some men it's a short period of inconvenience, for others a long and frustrating journey. The sections below describe techniques and technology for either curing incontinence or learning to live with it.

PADS AND ADULT DIAPERS

Once upon a time, incontinence wasn't acknowledged as an adult problem despite the fact that millions of men and women live with it. That's changing. Adult pads and diapers are now advertised on the evening news, and stores like Wal-Mart stock dozens of brands. Products for catching leaked urine come in all shapes and sizes, from complete diapers to small pads for lining the front of Jockey shorts. How do you find one that's right for you? "Start out with a small bag of the most absorbent, most body-covering ones you can find," suggests Bill, a sixty-six-year-old former lighting engineer. "If they don't fit or you don't need that much absorbency, you can move on to a smaller model without ending up with a month's supply of something you can't use."

Living with pads or diapers takes some adjustment. If you're retired and always at home, they don't pose that much of a problem. But if you work, travel, or just get out socially, you'll have to solve logistical problems like packing enough for the day and disposing of the soiled ones. Bill worked out a system of wrapping pads in individual sealable plastic bags. Whenever he needed to change, he would take out the dry pad and put the wet one in the watertight bag. That way he didn't have to worry about throwing it out in a friend's bathroom or in a public restroom.

Exercise and Behavior Modification
Like the ninety-eight-pound weakling turned beach strongman, an external sphincter can metamorphose into the single pumped-up muscle that controls urine flow. At the same time, simple tricks like drinking very little between dinner and bedtime or urinating on a schedule whether or not you really have to go can help minimize accidents and give you more control over urination.

The cornerstone of incontinence treatment is an exercise devised in the late 1940s by Dr. A. H. Kegel, a gynecologist. These simple exercises, still in widespread use today, strengthen the external sphincter and pelvic-floor muscles. When done properly, they help men overcome, or at least minimize, incontinence stemming from prostate cancer or its treatment. The beauty of these exercises is they require neither special equipment nor special clothing. They can be done while standing, driving a car, talking on the telephone, or lying on the couch. They take only a few minutes to do. They never make you break a sweat. What's more, they're invisible—you can do them at work surrounded by people and no one will be the wiser. "I started doing Kegel exercises while I still had my Foley in after the prostatectomy," says Eddie, a sixty-one-year-old bartender. "Then I would do them at work or when I was driving back and forth for the next few months. By my six-month postoperation anniversary I was completely dry."

Before you can strengthen the external sphincter, you have to find it. That's not easy, says Elizabeth Montgomery, an MGH urology nurse and incontinence specialist. Plenty of men do the exercises incorrectly and end up working their abdominal or gluteal (butt) muscles. Here are several different ways to identify the pelvic floor muscles that make up the external sphincter:

• Imagine you are in a crowded elevator and get the urge to pass gas. Squeeze the anal muscles that would spare your imaginary fellow passengers a malodorous ride. When you feel the anus pull inward and upward, you're also exercising the urinary sphincter.

• Stand naked in front of a full-length mirror. Contract your pelvic muscles until you find the ones that make your penis move up and down while the rest of you stays stationary.

• Sit or stand at the toilet and start to urinate, then try to hold back the stream. If you can reduce the flow by even a little, you're using the right muscles.

• If all else fails, wash your hands and insert one finger-tip into your anus. Do whatever it takes to contract the anus around your finger—the external urethral sphincter will contract at the same time, since they are part of the same muscle.

The exercise itself is stimple and straightforward. Contract the pelvic-floor muscles for several seconds, say a count of three to five, then relax them for the same time period. Repeat this tighten/relax cycle several times in a row. A man just healing from surgery might be able to tighten his sphincter and hold it for only three seconds a shot and do two or three in a row. Great—every little bit helps. Gradually increase both the duration of each contraction and the number you do each time. A reasonable daily goal? At least three sets of fifteen contractions, holding each one for ten seconds with a ten-second rest in between. Just for good measure, toss in a contraction or two every time a commercial comes on TV or whenever you stop at a red light. It also helps if you do some Kegel exercises standing, some sitting, and some lying down, since you'll eventually need to use them in each position.

You won't notice any improvement at first. A few days worth of Kegel exercises won't completely strengthen your external sphincter any more than a few days at the gym can build bulging biceps. But after two or three weeks of regular exercise, you should notice some improvement. Continued Kegel-ing usually brings even more obvious control.

Improper technique rarely leads to improved urine control, no matter how diligent you are about doing the exercises, and can make it worse. A common mistake is squeezing abdominal muscles rather than contracting the pelvic-floor muscles. This only serves to raise bladder pressure and actually increases the likelihood of incontinence. Place a hand on your belly when you do a contraction. If you feel muscles tighten or bunch up, you're working the wrong ones. Contracting the buttocks rather than pelvic-floor muscles will also be counterproductive. "And if you find yourself making faces or getting out of breath, then you probably aren't doing the exercises properly," says Ms. Montgomery. A urologist, urology nurse, or other incontinence specialist can help. Some use a biofeedback machine that actually measures the activity and strength of pelvic contractions to reinforce good technique.

Kegel exercises serve two purposes. They generally strengthen the external sphincter, making it a more powerful gatekeeper. Equally important, the exercises provide extra protection against stress incontinence. Just before you sneeze, laugh, or serve up a tennis ball, contract the external sphincter as if you were doing a Kegel exercise, and hold it for the duration of the sneeze or other stress. A conscious contraction or two is usually enough to offset increased pressure on the bladder and prevent urine loss.

With a little bit of luck and a lot of persistence, you will strengthen your external sphincter to the point where the pressure it exerts is greater than the pressure of a full bladder. That's continence. At that point you can gradually cut down on the number of Kegel contractions you do each day, since your normal activities probably give the sphincter plenty of exercise. If everything is fine, you can try stopping them altogether. And if you later notice you're leaking a drop or two of urine when you sneeze or climb stairs, go back and start Kegel-ing again.

Urge incontinence also responds to Kegel exercises plus some behavioral changes. This problem demands a mind-over-matter approach. The sudden, overwhelming feeling that you need to urinate often comes from a half-empty bladder that really doesn't need to be emptied. Believe it or not, this feeling can be controlled. As a small child you learned to associate a particular feeling with the need to go to the bathroom. Now you have to partially undo that learned behavior. When an urge strikes, contract your pelvic muscles, hard, several times in succession without fully relaxing in between. This is often enough to quell the urge. Sit quietly for a moment. Breathe deeply, or count backward from 100, until the urge has faded away. Only after calm prevails should you get up and walk, don't run, to the bathroom.

Drugs

When exercise and behavior modification don't work, or aren't quite enough to arrest incontinence, drugs can sometimes help. Stress incontinence responds to drugs that contract the pelvic-floor muscles. Examples include phenylpropanolamine (Dimetane), pseudoephedrine (found in Sudafed, Nyquil, and other over-the-counter cold remedies), and imipramine (Tofranil). Unfortunately, such drugs act on other muscles throughout the body. They can make your heart beat faster than normal, raise blood pressure, cause headaches, or disturb sleep. You and your clinician may have to experiment to find the right drug and the right dose for controlling incontinence without producing noticeable side effects.

Urge incontinence requires almost the opposite therapy. The drugs used to treat this condition relax the irritable smooth muscle surrounding the bladder and prevent the spasms that generate sudden urges to urinate. Several common medications include oxybutinin (Ditropan), flavoxate (Urispas), and nifedipine (Procardia). These, too, affect muscles throughout the body. Some men complain of a constantly dry mouth when taking these drugs, since they also relax the muscles that compress the salivary glands and pump saliva into the mouth. Other possible side effects include constipation, blurred vision, and dizziness upon standing up. Men who have glaucoma, or are at risk for it, usually aren't good candidates for anti-urge-incontinence drug therapy since most of these medications increase pressures inside the eye.

PENIS CLAMP

Near its tip, the urethra runs very close to the skin along the bottom side of the penis. Penis clamps (fig. 13.1) take advantage of this and mechanically compress the urethra, completely blocking urine flow. The clamps aren't as uncomfortable to wear as they are to look at or think about.

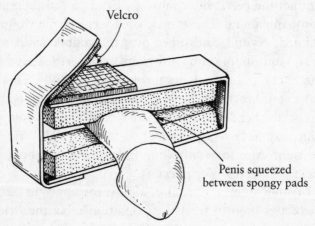

Velcro

Penis squeezed between spongy pads

Figure 13.1. *A Cunningham clamp squeezes the penis between soft, spongy pads. The pressure keeps the urethra shut, preventing urine from flowing out.*

Most are V-shaped and padded with soft foam. They fit just below the head of the penis. The urethra is so close to the surface here, and so compressible, only a small amount of pressure is needed to close it off. When it's time to urinate, a man merely releases the clamp and urine immediately begins to flow. A clamp can be arranged in boxer or Jockey shorts so it doesn't put an awkward lump behind a zipper.

A clamp offers a simple and effective solution for men plagued by moderate to severe incontinence. The main disadvantages? It can sometimes get uncomfortable, especially during vigorous activity. It clearly shows up under a tight bathing suit, and it is definitely noticeable in the locker room. In addition, it doesn't provide any protection when it is removed, say during sexual activity, a time you want maximum protection against incontinence.

CONDOM CATHETER

Like its namesake, this device (fig. 13.2) is rolled onto the penis. The tip ends in a small tube that connects to a collection bag. Urine leaving the penis collects in the catheter and drains into the bag, which can be strapped to the leg or hooked to the side of a bed or chair.

While a condom catheter keeps a man's clothing dry, it constantly bathes his penis in urine. A rash or irritation similar to diaper rash can develop unless the penis is carefully washed and dried several times a day. Men who use a condom catheter are also prone to developing irritating and painful bladder and urinary-tract infections. Some men find it difficult to keep the collection bag from sliding down the leg or leaking. As with the clamp, the condom catheter does nothing to strengthen muscles or improve continence and can't be used during sexual activity.

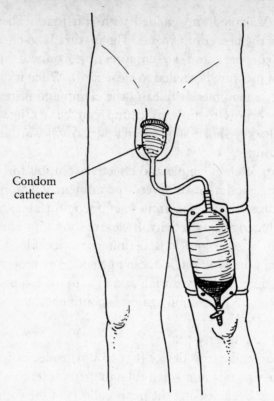

Condom
catheter

Figure 13.2. *A condom catheter is rolled onto the penis and held in place with a Velcro strip. Urine drains out a tube into a collection bag.*

ARTIFICIAL SPHINCTER

For severe incontinence that doesn't respond to exercise or medication, more and more men are turning to an artificial sphincter that is surgically implanted in the body. While several thousand men have opted for this solution over the last ten years, it isn't for everyone. A man with a hyperreflexive bladder—one prone to unexpected spasms—isn't a candidate, explains MGH urologist Dr.

Niall Heney. Nor is a man who also suffers from concurrent bladder cancer, recurrent urethral infections, or urethral strictures.

The device (fig. 13.3) consists of an expandable, fluid-filled cuff that is fitted around the urethra and a balloon-like reservoir placed inside the abdomen. Both are attached by flexible tubing to a pump the size of a plum pit fitted inside the scrotum. In the "on" position, fluid fills the cuff, pressing it into the base of the urethra much like a contracted sphincter muscle. Squeezing the pump several times draws fluid out of the cuff and sends it to the

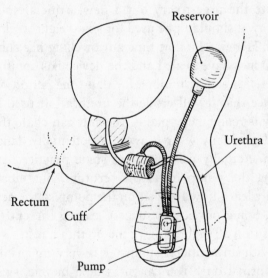

Figure 13.3. *An artificial sphincter is one way to stop incontinence. Most of the time, fluid fills the cuff, expanding it and making it squeeze the urethra shut. When it's time to void, a man presses the pump a few times. This transfers fluid from the cuff to the reservoir, deflating the cuff and allowing urine to pass through the urethra. After a few minutes, fluid returns to the cuff, once again blocking urine flow.*

reservoir. As the cuff drains and shrinks, the urethra expands and urine flows unimpeded past the sphincter. After two to three minutes, fluid automatically returns to the cuff, once again blocking the urine stream.

Implanting the device takes about two hours. The surgeon makes one incision in the scrotum for the pump. Through another incision, made between the scrotum and anus, he or she carefully wraps the cuff around the urethra, then places the reservoir into the abdomen. This is usually done under general anesthesia and should require no more than a one-day hospital stay. It can also be performed as day surgery, with no overnight stay.

Despite the urge to try out a new artificial sphincter right away, it shouldn't be used for six to eight weeks, cautions Dr. Heney. "By that time any swelling has subsided, all the tissues have healed and the device has comfortably seated itself. Leaving it alone for that time period reduces the chance that it will erode the urethra." If used before the body is ready, he explains, the cuff can chafe the urethra and gradually wear it away, a potentially dangerous situation. Actually using it takes some practice. At first, squeezing the pump hurts the scrotum, but most men eventually learn how to position the pump so the action is painless. Some physicians suggest leaving the cuff in the open position all night, to give the urethra a rest.

Life with an artificial sphincter is very much like life with a normal one. You can sit, ride a bicycle, swim, or make love and not realize it's there. "It saved my sanity and self-respect, and gave me back my life," says Ellis, a sixty-nine-year-old history professor. After radiation therapy and then cryosurgery, he found himself completely incontinent. "I stopped playing tennis, stopped meeting my friends for coffee every morning, stopped doing everything because I couldn't hold my water. Pads really limited my mobility and I didn't want to live the rest of my life with a catheter bag strapped to my leg," he says. After having an artificial sphincter implanted two years ago, he's back to his old routines.

Collagen Injections

A procedure that bulks up the top of the urethra aids some men and women whose incontinence stems from damage to the external sphincter. A natural protein called collagen, when injected on either side of the urethra, can thicken its walls until they almost touch. When done properly, this creates a movable, mechanical barrier to urine flow. High pressure inside the bladder temporarily forces aside the collagen bumps, opening the urethra for urination. As the bladder empties and the pressure inside the urethra falls, the collagen implants gradually come together again, virtually sealing the urethra shut. Most people require three or four injections spaced several weeks apart.

While this technique is highly successful for treating incontinence in women, for men with prostate-related incontinence the results have been only modestly encouraging. Only 25 to 30 percent of men who receive collagen injections stay completely dry. Urethral scars left over from prostate surgery or irradiation interfere with proper placement of the collagen and its ability to keep the urethra closed. The injections are also ineffective if an unstable or irritable bladder contributes to incontinence. Since many insurers consider collagen injections an experimental procedure, they don't generally cover it. At roughly $7,500 for three injection sessions, it makes for a pricey gamble if you have to pay for it yourself.

Impotence

This is the side effect of prostate-cancer treatment that men dread the most. "It's also the side effect men adapt to more readily than they initially might have believed," says MGH urologist Dr. Alex Althausen. "After they finish treatment and the future looks good, many men are simply happy to be alive and still with their family and friends. Sex often becomes less important after an experience like this."

It's still a difficult loss. For a man who equates sexuality with manhood, losing the ability to have sex represents a loss of manliness, a loss of identity, a diminishment of power. For any man it's an all-too-real manifestation of physical decline. It also represents an undeniable step toward old age that most of us would rather put off as long as possible. Even men who haven't had sex in years mourn the passing of their erections. "I haven't been with a woman since my wife died almost fifteen years ago, and don't ever expect to be with another. But the *idea* that I can't make love again really makes me mad sometimes," says Abe, an eighty-one-year-old former truck dispatcher.

Treatment for prostate cancer can cause erectile dysfunction (the medical term for impotence) in several ways. Surgery can cut or damage the nerves responsible for controlling penile blood vessels, the anatomic players that actually create an erection. Radiation can kill these nerve cells, just as it kills nearby tumor cells. Orchiectomy or hormone therapy blocks the production or action of testosterone, a crucial requirement for both normal erections and sex drive. And more often than most men would like to admit, impotence may have been just around the corner even without treatment. In a survey of 1,200 randomly selected Massachusetts men, investigators from the New England Research Institute documented what experts had long known—the incidence of impotence increases with age and poor health. Among forty-year-old men in the survey, about 20 percent reported moderate impotence and 5 percent complete impotence. For seventy-year-olds, the rates rose to 35 percent and 15 percent. Over all age categories, 43 percent of smokers who were being treated for heart disease reported being completely impotent, compared to 5 percent of nonsmokers without heart disease.

Accurate or realistic numbers on erectile problems following prostate-cancer treatment are hard to pin down. Impotence is not a subject that most men, and that includes male physicians, talk about openly. It's not uncommon for the discussion to run two brief sentences. "How are you doing sexually, Mr. Jones?" "I'm doing okay, Doc." In such a discussion, "okay" could mean everything from normal erections to soft erections or no erections at all but I'd rather not talk about it. Men can be plain old embarrassed to tell another man—physician or not—they are impotent. Another factor complicating the picture is that researchers don't always define or measure potency after surgery or radiation the same way. In some studies it may involve merely a single question: Do you have erections? Others phrase it more specifically: Do you have erections firm enough to achieve penetration, or have you and your partner had satisfactory sexual intercourse in the last month? Such different questions yield very different numbers. Finally, most of the studies reported in the medical literature come from the country's best practitioners and prostate experts. Most of them see hundreds of men with prostate cancer a year, and are often able to select the patients they choose to treat. Thus the men involved in studies reported in the medical literature aren't necessarily a representative sample of the average American man with prostate cancer.

That said, the most often-quoted numbers for posttreatment potency are these: Following a nerve-sparing prostatectomy, approximately 70 percent of men regain some erectile function within twelve months. Following radiation therapy, approximately 50 percent to 60 percent of men retain erectile function two years or longer after treatment. The *real* numbers are probably somewhat lower, if the results from an ongoing study at the Dana Farber Cancer Institute in Boston are any indication. The researchers asked 192 men treated in the Boston area for prostate cancer to fill out a long questionnaire regarding the side effects of surgery or radiation. At twelve months posttreatment, only 23 percent of men who chose a radical prostatectomy reported having an erection in the previous four weeks. Put another way, 77 percent were impotent. For those who had chosen radiation therapy, 59 percent said they had recently experienced an erection. "If we were to follow up on these same men at three years after treatment, we think it might be around 50-percent potency in both groups since it can take that long for impotence to develop after radiation therapy and that long for erectile function to return after surgery," says lead investigator Dr. James Talcott.

The odds of becoming impotent after prostate cancer treatment depend on several factors. The surgeon's or radiotherapist's skill is of utmost importance. Treatment at the hands of an experienced, careful practitioner leads to fewer side effects of all types. A man's health and prior sexual function also play a large role. Younger men fare better than older men. Men who regularly engaged in sexual activity before treatment tend to have a better chance of retaining sexual function than those who had previously given up on sex. Otherwise healthy men also fare better than their less healthy counterparts, since circulatory problems, diabetes, cigarette smoking, and depression all contribute to impotence.

A warning here: Even for the healthiest, most sexually active men, posttreatment erections don't always compare to pretreatment erections. More often than not, erections after surgery or radiation therapy tend to be more difficult to initiate, softer, and quicker to fade without direct stimulation. Radiation therapy invariably damages some nerves needed for proper erectile function, and a nerve-sparing prostatectomy may only spare the nerves on one side of the prostate. Stress of treatment, worries about recurrence, and the flood of life changes that often accompany cancer also contribute to these changes.

Do softer erections, or none at all, mean the death of sex? Not unless you let them. The penis's sensory nerves don't come anywhere near the prostate and aren't affected by treatment—even a limp penis can feel a touch, a stroke. With enough stimulation, a man can have a perfectly pleasurable orgasm without an erection. Orgasms following prostatectomy and radiation therapy, however, are invariably dry—no semen shoots out of the penis. (Such dry ejaculations also mean that a man is unable to father a child.) Despite these changes, many couples continue to have a healthy, happy, and active sex life in spite of impotence. But it takes patience, a sense of humor, the openness to explore, and a lot of talking.

Anatomy

The prostate's main function relates to reproduction. It manufactures a host of proteins, sugars, and other substances that feed and protect sperm on their journey from penis to fallopian tubes. A ripple of muscular contractions during orgasm propels accumulated prostate fluid into the urethra just in time to meet sperm and other fluids from the seminal vesicles. Urethral contractions shoot this mixture, called semen, out of the penis.

The prostate itself neither initiates nor maintains erections. Those tasks belong to the testes, to nerves that just happen to use the prostate for support as they travel from spinal cord to penis, and to the penis itself. The testes make testosterone, often called the male hormone even though women also manufacture small amounts of it. Testosterone somehow controls the sex drive by floating through the bloodstream and interacting with cells in the hypothalamus, a small part of the brain stem that controls functions like eating, sleeping, breathing, and reproduction. Without testosterone, the sex drive fades and erections no longer happen, either spontaneously or with assistance.

The "erection" signal begins in the brain, triggered by a touch, a fantasy, a smell or sound or sight. It travels down the spinal cord and then through a pair of smaller nerves to the penis. For years urologists believed these nerves ran *through* the prostate on their way to the penis, and that's why prostatectomy destroyed the ability to have an erection. It wasn't until the late 1970s that Dr. Patrick Walsh, chief of urology at Johns Hopkins, and Dr. Pieter Donker, a retired professor of urology in the Netherlands, discovered that these nerves ran along either side of the prostate capsule, and merely used the gland for support on their way to the penis. (This led Walsh to develop the nerve-sparing prostatectomy now practiced around the country.)

A penis is composed of three soft, spongy cylinders filled with a network of blood vessels and muscle. The lower cylinder, or corpus spongiosum, carries the urethra and some blood vessels. The other two cylinders, the paired corpora cavernosa, are what actually expand and stiffen. During sexual arousal, nerves send a "relax" signal to small arteries inside the corpora cavernosa. Blood flow into the relaxed arteries increases dramatically. All this extra blood expands the spongy muscle, and this stiffens the penis. The expanding tissue also compresses veins that normally drain blood out of the corpora cavernosae, trapping blood inside the penis. Eventually, blood pressure inside the engorged organ becomes so high that no more blood can enter.

Distraction, lack of stimulation, and orgasm all have the opposite effect. Different nerves send a "contract" signal. The arteries narrow, slowing blood flow into the penis. As spongy muscle begins constricting, it no longer compresses the veins, thus allowing blood to flow away from the penis faster and faster. The erection fades in a process called detumescence.

Intact nerves, working blood vessels, adequate blood flow, and enough testosterone are all required for an erection. Problems with any one component can lead to impotence. Men with poor circulation due to heart disease or smoking, for example, often suffer from impotence. Those with degenerative nerve disease often lose the ability to have erections. And men with very low levels of testosterone often lose interest in sex as well as their capacity for erections.

How Treatment Causes Impotence

Surgery causes impotence by injuring nerves that carry the erection signal and run along the sides of the prostate. They don't grow back after this. In the early days of prostatectomy, surgeons removed the entire gland and a generous zone of tissue around it. They did this to increase the odds they removed all the malignant cells. This zone, or margin, of tissue invariably included the neurovascular bundles and thus left virtually all men impotent. The nerve-sparing prostatectomy developed in the 1980s takes a more conservative approach when possible. The surgeon still removes the entire gland, but tries to leave the neurovascular bundles intact if the tumor does not appear to come near them. While such a strategy appears to be effective, "it goes against the most common tenet surgeons hold for cancer operations—take as wide a margin of tissue as possible," points out Dr. Heney. It's impossible for your urologist to know how extensive the tumor is, or if it involves the nerves, before beginning the operation. So there's no way to guarantee potency beforehand. Before agreeing to the operation, you should know that your surgeon will remove whatever tissue is needed to eradicate the tumor, even if that means taking the nerves that control erections.

Radiation therapy also causes impotence. Since the neurovascular bundles straddle the prostate, it's impossible to shield them from the radiation. High-energy beams zipping through the nerve cells disrupt important enzymes, kill cells, and introduce tiny errors into the genetic material. If enough damage accumulates, nerve fibers can die. This doesn't necessarily happen right away; it can take up to two to three years. And sometimes it doesn't happen at all, since otherwise healthy cells can survive radiation's immediate effects and repair the damage while tumor cells usually cannot.

Hormone therapy leaves nerves and blood vessels perfectly intact, yet leads to impotence far more often than either surgery or radiation therapy. That's because it disrupts the natural hormone cycle that drives sexual function in men, from sparking the desire for sex to triggering and maintaining an erection. Normally, tiny testosterone molecules produced in the testes sidle into the brain. They mysteriously drum up interest in sex, both mentally and physically. When testosterone levels plummet well below normal, after castration or with an LHRH agonist drug, so does the sex drive and the capacity for erections. A minority of men, however, somehow remain sexually interested and active even without much testosterone circulating through the bloodstream.

Taking Action

Finding out you have prostate cancer, then putting up with the indignities of diagnosis and treatment, is bad enough. Impotence adds insult to injury. This unwanted but often unavoidable condition generates different feelings in men. Some get angry, others depressed. Some feel sad, others embarrassed. Some accept it as part of growing older, though perhaps come a tad early, others fight it with all the weapons of modern medicine.

Impotence is generally a shared condition—with a long-time partner, a new paramour, or future romantic or sexual interest. And that means it's not just your problem, one you must solve by yourself. Ignoring your partner's opinions or wishes could lead to discord and resentment.

Joseph, a sixty-eight-year-old retired machinist, decided to have a penile implant after a radical prostatectomy left him impotent: "I felt kind of old, and not being able to have an erection in bed made things even worse. I thought an implant would help. But my wife really hates it because she says it's unnatural. So it's actually caused more problems than we had before."

Joseph's unspoken message is this: Don't assume you know what your partner wants. Most would probably echo this sentiment from sixty-nine-year-old Sylvia. She runs a fabric store with her husband, who had a prostatectomy two years ago: "As long as he's there to talk with me, read the paper with me, go to sleep and wake up with me, that's all I want. As long as he's here with me, sex isn't important."

That's not to say your partner isn't interested in continuing the sexual side of your relationship, assuming you had one before starting the battle against prostate cancer. The question often becomes whether or not to use technology to reestablish sexual activity. Some couples adapt their lovemaking so it doesn't require an erect penis. Others want, or need, an erection as part of their sexual repertoire.

Couples who talk openly and honestly about everything—sex included—will take this topic in stride. New couples, or those who don't always communicate well, might need some help. Try meeting with a social worker or therapist, especially one who works with couples on sexuality issues. If one isn't available at your local hospital, call or write the American Association of Sex Educators, Counselors and Therapists (see Resources) for a list of certified counselors in your area.

Two other resources may give you and your partner

more information and better ways to talk about this difficult subject. The Impotence Institute of America (see Resources) has produced an excellent videotape and publishes a newsletter about impotence. It also sponsors regular Impotents Anonymous meetings in major cities around the country. These offer a source of information and a forum for discussion with other men in the same boat. A prostate-cancer support group such as Us-Too or Man-to-Man (see Resources) can also give you personal help. The men and their partners who attend these groups are intimately familiar with your dilemma and can give you down-to-earth advice and encouragement.

The product of your soul-searching and conversations with your partner will be some decision on what to do about impotence. Some couples choose to live with it, either because sex hadn't been an important part of their relationship for some time, or because they want to see how satisfying they can make the alternatives. Other couples decide to explore aids such as those described below.

Injection Technique

You're probably thinking, "No way would I ever stick a needle into my penis!" But the thousands of men who use this technique say it is neither bizarre nor painful. It requires a tiny needle and a watery mixture of drugs, usually some combination of papaverine, phentolamine, or prostaglandin E. You make the injection about halfway down one side of the penis. The skin here, while exquisitely sensitive to touch and sexual stimulation, doesn't have many pain receptors. The needle stick feels like a mosquito bite. As the drugs spread throughout the penis, they relax small arteries in the two corpora cavernosae, the cylinders filled with spongy muscle tissue. In five to ten minutes blood begins to flow into the relaxed, expanded arteries, swelling the spongy tissue and blocking off veins that carry blood away. It's the exact same mechanism that creates a natural erection, except these are triggered by a drug rather than a nerve impulse. The erection lasts from thirty minutes to two hours. In some men it begins to fade soon after orgasm, while in others it lasts until the drugs wear off.

All men require a test run or two in their physician's office to practice the injection technique and determine the right dose. Some men are supersensitive to these drugs and a small dose can cause priapism, says William Casey, an MGH urology nurse who teaches men to use the injection technique. Priapism is basically an erection that won't go away after two hours. This condition is both painful and potentially harmful to the penis. It can be reversed by injecting into the penis a drug that constricts blood vessels. If an injection-induced erection won't subside, call your physician immediately.

An erection produced by the injection technique resembles a natural erection in every way. It is firm, warm, and requires no accessories or devices to maintain. There are, however, several limitations, points out Mr. Casey. It can't be used whenever you get the urge. A man must *never* inject himself twice in one day, or even on consecutive days. Three times a week should be the maximum. More than this can damage the entire erectile mechanism. In addition, some men find that the injections lead to bruising outside the penis or scarring inside. The drugs themselves can sometimes depress liver function. The technique itself can be tricky, requiring good eyesight, good manual dexterity, and no squeamishness about needles. Furthermore, the drugs must be kept refrigerated, which complicates traveling.

The injection therapy isn't exactly cheap. It costs somewhere between $5 and $15 per injection, depending on the mixture of drugs you need and how much your pharmacy charges for them. And they usually aren't covered by Medicare.

Vacuum-Assisted Devices

Another popular and effective technique for creating an erection uses what's called a vacuum device or vacuum erection device. These relatively simple pumps (fig. 13.4) put the "Nature abhors a vacuum" principle to work. By lowering the air pressure around a man's penis, they allow blood vessels to expand. Extra blood flows into the enlarged penile blood vessels and expands the organ, mimicking the action of a normal erection.

The device consists of a hard, plastic cylinder that's open at the bottom and connected to a mechanism for removing air at the top. You lubricate your penis and slip it into a condom-shaped space inside the cylinder, then press the open end tightly against your scrotum and lower abdomen. The lubricant and pressure help form an airtight seal. Once everything is in place you pump air out of the cylinder. It may take five minutes or so for an erection to begin rising. After the cylinder is removed, you roll a rubber retention ring down to the base of the penis. This rubber band–like ring compresses blood vessels, trapping the erection-causing blood in the penis. The erection lasts until the ring is removed.

Unlike the injection technique, a man can use a vacuum erection device as often as he wants, says Mr. Casey. It's

Vacuum Device

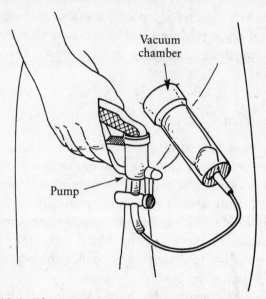

Vacuum
chamber

Pump

Figure 13.4. *Thousands of men use vacuum devices to get an erection. The vacuum chamber is fitted onto the penis and pressed snugly against the pubis. Operating the pump pulls air out of the chamber, allowing blood to rush into the penis. Once a satisfactory erection has arisen, a rubber ring is rolled down to the base of the penis and the chamber is removed. This maintains the erection by preventing blood from leaving the penis.*

also portable, needn't be refrigerated, and doesn't interfere with liver function. In the long run it is also less expensive—high-quality devices cost around $400, and Medicare usually picks up 80 percent of that cost as long as it has been prescribed by a physician.

Vacuum erection devices aren't for everyone. Men who

have high blood pressure or those taking anticoagulation medications usually aren't candidates because the device can cause bleeding around the penis. Some men try the device but stop using it for several reasons. Some find the vacuum sensation painful, or experience temporary swelling. The retention ring bothers some men and their partners. The quality of vacuum erections is another issue. They begin warm, but gradually cool since no blood circulates through the penis. And the shaft below the band can remain soft, making an erection somewhat floppy or hard to control. Finally, creating the erection takes several minutes, and is usually done just before intercourse. So it can interrupt lovemaking, or introduce a mechanical aspect that some couples find intrusive or less than romantic. The trick, suggests Mr. Casey, is incorporating the device into the whole ritual of lovemaking. While it may seem weird at first, it can become a mutually enjoyed part of the activity.

Penile Implants

Throughout this century, men and their physicians have experimented with surgically implanting stiff rods of rib cartilage or synthetic material into the penis for erectile support. Most failed. But over the past twenty years or so, two basic designs have become widely accepted. One uses a flexible but rigid rod, the other an inflatable device.

A semirigid prosthesis is a rod made of inert silicone implanted inside the penis (fig 13.5). This requires an hour-long operation during which the pencil-thin rod is positioned above the urethra. This yields a penis that is permanently stiff. Though the erection is sufficiently hard for penetration, it gets neither longer nor wider during sexual activity. A penis with a semirigid prosthesis can be pressed against the body or pointed downward along the upper thigh. In this way it can be effectively concealed inside boxer shorts. "No one can tell that I have anything I wasn't born with," says Norman, a sixty-three-year-old auto mechanic. He says he and his wife are both pleased with the implant, but admits he's a bit more private in the locker room now when he goes to the Y for his twice-weekly swim.

The increasingly popular inflatable prosthesis allows for erections on demand. One model consists of two collapsible, fluid-filled cylinders implanted into the shaft of the penis, a fluid reservoir tucked into the abdomen and a small pump placed in the scrotum (fig. 13.5). In the flaccid state, all the fluid sits in the reservoir. To create an erection, a man squeezes the pump several times, transferring fluid from the reservoir to the cylinders. This hydraulic action telescopes them outward, elongating the penis and also increasing its diameter. Detumescence is accomplished by pressing the pump's release valve, which drains fluid from the cylinders and returns it to the reservoir.

A somewhat simpler inflatable prosthesis consists of two interlocking, fluid-filled hydraulic cylinders placed inside the shaft of the penis. Squeezing the pump located on the end of one cylinder just beneath the glans, or head, of the penis redistributes the fluid and stiffens the penis. While this kind of implant doesn't yield the same noticeable increase in length or girth as its three-piece cousin, it still yields a workable erection.

Penile implants offer men a level of control and subtlety they don't have with the injection technique or vacuum erection device. While some manipulation is still necessary, creating an erection isn't nearly as obvious. What's

Penile Implants

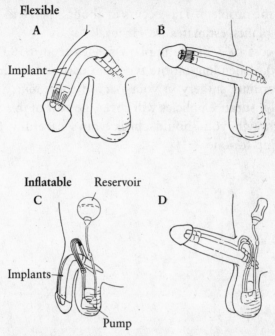

Figure 13.5. *There are two main types of penile implants. Flexible implants are permanently rigid, and can be positioned down along the leg (A) or outward for sexual activity (B). Inflatable implants work much like artificial sphincters. A pump in the scrotum is used to move fluid from a reservoir (C) into the prosthesis. As it fills with fluid, it lengthens and creates an erection (D). Later, the pump is used to reverse the process.*

more, implants don't place a limit on the number of erections a man can have each day, nor do they cause any bruising, scarring, bleeding, or problems with liver function. One drawback is that an implant requires a surgical procedure, with its attendant risks from anesthesia or infection. Another is that the erection is cool and, to some men and their partners, "unlifelike." Finally, inflatable implants sometimes fail, requiring a second operation to take care of the problem. This occurs in about 3 percent of men with implants, estimates Dr. Heney.

The cost of a penile implant ranges from $10,000 to $20,000, depending on the type you choose and the cost of performing surgery in your part of the country. Most medical insurance policies will cover the cost of this procedure, though you should check yours carefully before signing up for one.

14

Coping with Pain

Though prostate cancer begins silently and completely unnoticed, it can evolve into a very painful disease. A tumor that distorts and inflames the prostate gland or compresses nearby nerves can produce painful sensations in the urethra, rectum, and lower abdomen. Metastases to pelvic bones or the spine generate back or leg pain often intensified by movement. Distant spread to the skull can produce intense headaches or sinus pain while metastases to arm, leg, or rib bones may cause painful fractures. Not only is pain a regular presence for the majority of men with advanced or metastatic prostate cancer, it's the kind of symptom that can't be ignored. Sure, many men grit their teeth, try to will away pain, and pretend everything is fine. But when it permeates every telephone call, backswing, climb up the stairs, or family dinner, it's downright unhealthy. The newest research suggests that chronic pain increases stress, weakens the immune system, and leads to depression, all of which make one more susceptible to cancer's spread and less able to tolerate treatment.

Four things you should know about pain:

- Modern therapies let you control pain without being drugged into drowsiness or a stupor.
- It is far easier to prevent pain, or to control it while still mild, than it is to turn off intense pain.
- Pain only gets worse if you ignore it.
- Real men feel pain, admit they hurt, and do something about it.

No one need live with pain. "We have an impressive array of drugs and dosing strategies that allow people with chronic pain to live comfortable, active lives," says Dr. David Borsook, director of the MGH Pain Center.

This hasn't always been the case. Until recently, people with advanced cancer often suffered terribly. Not through any fault of their own. Researchers and patient advocates pointed the finger at physicians who traditionally under-treated pain—partly out of fear their patients would become addicted to narcotics, partly because they thought it necessary to hold something in reserve for when pain intensified. In a 1988 *Newsweek* interview, the former director of the National Institute on Drug Abuse, Dr. Charles Schuster, blasted physicians for their timidity in this area. "The way we treat cancer pain borders on a national disgrace," he said.

But over the last few years, advocacy groups and enlightened physicians have turned the spotlight on cancer pain. Thanks to their efforts, comfort and quality of life are now the key goals of treatment. More and more, pain is seen as a debilitating foe and treated as aggressively as the cancer that generates it. In 1994, a panel of experts cochaired by Dr. Daniel Carr, former director of the MGH Pain Center, published national practice guidelines for treating cancer pain.[1] In a nutshell, the guidelines say this: "Whenever pain is present, clinicians should provide optimal pain relief by routinely assessing pain and treating it." (To order a free copy of the guidelines, see Resources.)

Some pains are easy to eliminate, others aren't. If you and your physician can't manage yours, you might want to seek out a specialist. Most hospitals have one or more pain experts; some, like MGH, have an entire clinic devoted to pain control. In addition, more than thirty states have developed cancer-pain initiatives, most of them based on pioneering work from the Wisconsin Cancer Pain Initiative (see Resources).

What Is Pain and How Is It Treated?

When body tissues are sliced, crushed, stretched, twisted, or otherwise damaged, cells release chemicals that act as potent messengers. These chemicals, called prostaglandins, trigger specialized nerve cells to send signals to the spinal cord and brain. We interpret these signals as pain. Prostaglandins also make nearby cells extrasensitive to painful stimuli—that's why even the uninjured tissue near an elbow scrape or finger gouge is so tender.

Cancer triggers all sorts of pain receptors. Tumor growth stretches and distorts tissues, releasing a steady stream of prostaglandins. Swollen tissues or growing tumors sometimes compress nearby nerves, setting off a cascade of pain signals to the brain. Bony metastatic tumors

[1] A. Jacox et al., *Management of Cancer Pain*, AHCPR Publication no. 94-0592 (Washington: Agency for Health Care Policy Research, 1994).

dramatically increase the pressure inside bones, rupturing some cells and squeezing others aside. The end result of all this is pain—steady throbbing, sharp stabs, dull constant aches, burning, or itching.

"Pain associated with advanced prostate cancer poses a real problem," says Dr. Borsook. "This is a slow-growing cancer, so men often live with it and the pain it produces for a long time." The most difficult challenge is defusing bone pain. For some reason, malignant cells that escape a prostate tumor migrate to bones around the body, especially those in the pelvis and spine. Sometimes these tumors seem to radiate pain, even those that are too small to see on a bone scan or other diagnostic test. Fortunately, drugs or radiation can keep it in check.

There are several avenues to halting cancer pain. Surgically removing a tumor or shrinking it with radiation or hormone therapy takes the pressure off compressed nerves and halts prostaglandin production. A class of drugs known as nonsteroidal anti-inflammatory drugs (NSAIDs) prevent cells from assembling prostaglandins. It's also possible to block transmission of pain signals. Morphine and other narcotics somehow render nerves unable to send this message, or they interfere with the brain's ability to interpret it. Selectively severing nerves can accomplish the same goal. Finally, some people find relief in nonmedical alternatives such as meditation, hypnosis, biofeedback, and acupuncture.

The whole key to comfort is this: Fight pain as soon as it appears—even before it appears, if possible—and do whatever it takes to make it vanish. That strategy makes good medical sense. As mentioned earlier, the chemical events occurring inside the body that make you feel pain simultaneously reduce your threshold for pain. In other words, pain makes you more sensitive to further pain, and it takes higher doses of drugs to stop it.

Even more important, preventing pain also makes perfect sense for your health and well-being. Chronic pain does more than simply hurt. It magnifies the stress you're already under because of the cancer itself. More stress causes the body to overproduce stress hormones, which make the heart beat faster, increase blood sugar, depress appetite, and disrupt sleep habits. Ultimately this magnifies any cancer-caused debilitation. In a vicious cycle it also lowers your tolerance for pain. Over time, chronic pain and stress also weaken the immune response and make it harder for the body to fight the spread of cancer. Unrelieved pain also drives some people to the brink of depression, prompting them to give up and stop treatment, hoping that a quick death will bring it to an end.

Proper pain-control measures can eliminate these extra stresses, stop unnecessary suffering, and give you back an enjoyable, productive life. They will also give your family or loved ones important emotional relief—few things are as difficult as watching someone you care for struggle with pain. "That was the worst part," says seventy-year-old Jane, whose husband died after a long battle with metastatic prostate cancer. "He hurt so much and nothing the doctors did, or nothing I did, seemed to help."

The sections below describe state-of-the-art approaches to controlling pain resulting from advanced prostate cancer.

Hormone Therapy

For men with advanced prostate cancer, the first defense against pain entails shrinking local, regional, or metastatic tumors. This is primarily done with hormone therapy, though radiation (see page 227) and chemotherapy (see page 236) are also options. Hormone therapy aims to reduce the amount of testosterone circulating in the bloodstream. Without this hormone, prostate-derived tumors tend to stop growing and may shrivel up, reducing the pressure inside bones or pulling tissue away from nerves.

There are two basic ways to lower testosterone levels. Drugs such as estrogen or LHRH agonists stop the testes from making and secreting testosterone. Or an operation called orchiectomy removes the testes and with them the body's ability to manufacture this hormone. *Warning*: If your choice of hormone therapy is an LHRH agonist like leuprolide (Lupron) or goserelin (Zoladex), and you are already experiencing some pain, make sure your physician also has you take an antiandrogen. Lupron and Zoladex temporarily increase testosterone levels and can thus swell tumors and dramatically increase pain or slow urine flow. Antiandrogens such as flutamide (Eulexin) or bicalutamide (Casodex) prevent any circulating testosterone from oozing inside cells and thus block its ability to stimulate cell growth and division. An antiandrogen isn't needed with an orchiectomy, since the testosterone-making machinery has been removed.

About 80 percent of men initially respond to hormone therapy. But over time its ability to control the spread of prostate cancer, and thus pain, diminishes. Eventually, other therapies are needed. The 20 percent of men with hormone-insensitive prostate cancer must turn immediately to other measures for dealing with pain.

Painkillers

You've probably been using drugs to stop simple aches and pains for years. Some of these same drugs play a role in warding off prostate-cancer pain, though the doses may be higher.

Men have two main fears when it comes to taking painkilling drugs: Will I become so sedated I can't function? Will I become addicted to these drugs? The answer to both is a resounding *no*. New drugs and dosing schemes can eliminate drowsiness while adequately quelling pain. And addiction just isn't an issue. Researchers at the Medical College of Wisconsin, one of the country's leaders in cancer-pain treatment, reviewed more than 15,000 patients taking narcotic drugs for pain. They found only three with signs of drug dependence. Addiction is the compulsive use of drugs for pleasure—pain clearly doesn't fall into that category.

The World Health Organization has established a "three-step ladder" for treating pain that has become standard procedure in the United States and around the world. It starts with over-the-counter drugs like aspirin and ibuprofen on the lowest rung and gradually moves up to stronger medications like codeine and morphine. The trick is *preventing* pain rather than trying to beat it down once it appears.

To accomplish this preventive strike, take your pain medication on a prearranged schedule, even if you aren't hurting. If, now and then, pain "breaks through" and appears between scheduled doses, take what specialists call a rescue dose. How do you and your physician determine the best schedule and amount of medication to take? "The right dose is how much you need to get rid of pain," says Dr. Borsook.

The World Health Organization ladder looks like this:

Step 1: Nonsteroidal anti-inflammatory agents, or NSAIDs, and nonnarcotic analgesics form the first rung of the painkiller ladder. Aspirin, acetominophen (Tylenol), and ibuprofen (Motrin, Advil, Nuprin, and others) all fit into this category. If your physician prescribes one of these for intense pain, don't immediately assume he or she isn't taking you seriously. The right dose of some over-the-counter drugs can be as effective as morphine. NSAIDs are particularly effective against bone pain because they somehow slow metastatic prostate cancer's ability to destroy normal bone tissue. They also reduce local inflammation and inhibit the synthesis of prostaglandins, compounds that make pain receptors extrasensitive.

You'll generally be started on a low dose of an NSAID, which should be taken with food or just after a meal or snack. It may take a day or two before the full effects are felt, so give the drugs a chance to work. But if they clearly aren't taking care of pain, let your physician know right away. Don't wait a week or month until your next visit. And don't increase the daily dose on your own, since these drugs can potentially damage the kidneys or liver. Your physician should either increase the dose or switch you to another NSAID, since some men respond to one but not another. For your part, take the drug at the prescribed intervals throughout the day, even if you aren't hurting when it's time for the next dose. As mentioned before, it requires less medication to prevent pain from returning than it does to banish it once it arrives.

Sometimes NSAIDs can't keep up as pain escalates. They have "ceiling doses" above which you get no extra pain relief, only more side effects. These side effects are fairly limited, and affect a minority of men. NSAIDs can upset the stomach, and may worsen any preexisting kidney problems. They may also make some men a bit depressed or unable to sleep well at night, says Dr. Borsook. An antidepressant or sleeping pill can counter these, if needed.

Step 2: Mild or weak opioids can be added to NSAIDs for more pain relief. These, too, are common drugs you might have had prescribed after a minor operation or a wisdom-tooth extraction. Examples include codeine, which is often combined with aspirin or acetaminophen (Tylenol plus codeine), propoxyphene (Darvon), oxycodone (Percodan, Percocet), and others. Most are available in tablet or liquid form. Here again you want to take each dose on schedule, just before pain returns. As with NSAIDs, if the prescribed dose isn't working, ask your doctor or nurse to either adjust the dosage or switch you to another kind.

Step 3: Strong opioids represent the next stage of pain control if NSAIDs and weak opioids don't work. Morphine is the "gold standard" by which all other pain-control efforts are measured. Alternatives exist, primarily for men who cannot tolerate morphine. These include fentanyl, methadone, and others. With strong opioids, no ceiling dose exists—increasing the dose always brings more relief. But it also brings more side effects, and at some point these begin to outweigh the drug's beneficial effects.

The most common side effects are drowsiness, constipation, and nausea, followed by nightmares or hallucinations and trouble urinating. Taking a lower dose, as long as it still relieves pain, may be enough to dispel drowsiness. A mild stimulant like caffeine can counteract opioid sedation. And a group of researchers from Edmonton

General Hospital in Canada have strong evidence to show that the drug methylphenidate (Ritalin), often used to calm hyperactive children, not only perks up people taking strong opioids like morphine but also may add to the drug's painkilling activity. Dietary changes can usually counteract constipation. Drink as much liquid as you can, preferably beverages that contain neither alcohol nor caffeine. High-fiber foods or a stool-softening laxative also help.

Dr. Borsook adds a *Step 4* to the WHO ladder: Even the strongest opioids can lose their punch against cancer pain. When that happens, these drugs can be administered in novel ways that boost their painkilling power. The powerful opioid fentanyl, for example, can be delivered continuously through a patch worn on the skin for three days at a time. Two types of portable pumps easily concealed under clothing have also been a boon to men with prostate cancer pain. One pump, called the patient-controlled analgesia (PCA) pump, delivers a preset dose of a painkilling drug whenever you press a small button. A tiny computer keeps track to make sure you don't accidentally overdose yourself. The other delivers a continuous infusion of painkiller through a small needle placed under the skin.

Other Medical Therapies

Injections of radioactive strontium-89 were recently approved by the Food and Drug Administration as a nonnarcotic treatment for bone pain. This substance, sold as Metastron, mimics calcium in the body and gets incorporated into bones. Once there, it emits high-energy radiation that kills nearby tumor cells. Metastron doesn't completely destroy bone tumors, which would be a big step toward curing metastatic prostate cancer. But it does make them smaller and less painful. In clinical trials, Metastron helped control pain in 70 percent of men with bone metastases; 20 percent of them said it made their pain disappear. Since Metastron can't tell one cell from another, it also kills off bone-marrow cells that manufacture crucial blood components, platelets and white blood cells. Too few white blood cells may compromise the body's ability to fight infection, while too few platelets in circulation can interfere with the blood's clotting ability. This side effect usually limits Metastron's use to men in the terminal stage of their disease.

The drug is usually administered as a single injection in a doctor's office or medical center clinic. It begins to work in a week or so, after which it's possible to begin tapering off daily doses of painkillers. The effects last anywhere from three to six months, and the treatment can be repeated. Injections of Metastron, or a similar drug called samarium-103 now under investigation, don't make you radioactive. You don't need lead-lined clothes to hug your partner, sit next to a business associate, or hold a grandchild on your lap. If you are sexually active, use a condom for the first week, just as a precaution against any minuscule amounts of radioactivity your semen might carry. And incontinent men should consider a catheter for the first week or so to prevent contaminating their clothing or bedding. In any case the amount of radioactivity released in semen, urine, feces, or blood is exceedingly small and unlikely to harm anyone.

External radiation also plays a role in pain control. Doses of radiation directed at painful bone metastases can halt tumor growth, at least temporarily. This approach both controls pain and helps prevent cancer-related fractures. It cannot, however, be repeated once pain returns to the same spot—one course of radiation, which may involve several separate treatments, is all that a single area can handle.

A rather drastic procedure called hemibody radiation is sometimes used when other treatments fail to control pain caused by widespread bone metastases. This is a single dose of radiation directed over half the body. If pain persists, the other half can be irradiated after a three-week interval. In several studies, this technique provides pain relief in about 48 hours for 50 percent of the men who try it; it takes longer in others. This much radiation, about three times more than given to the prostate during any single treatment, destroys a fair amount of bone marrow and may hamper the body's infection-fighting ability. Hemibody radiation can control pain for several months, often long enough to give a man with advanced prostate cancer some pain-free time during the final stage of his illness.

Drugs called *diphosphonates* may also be used to fight uncontrollable bone pain. The compounds etidronate and pamidronate block the metabolic activity of bone cells called osteoclasts, and thus prevent tumors from dissolving bone tissue and using the raw materials for their own growth.

Chemotherapy, described in Chapter 12, is also an avenue for alleviating prostate-cancer pain. So far, though, the results haven't been encouraging enough to make them a standard option for all men.

If all other methods fail, surgical procedures can sometimes help control pain. In a *rhizotomy*, a surgeon cuts nerves that carry pain signals from one part of the body to the spinal cord. A more radical version of this is called a *cordotomy*, in which bundles of nerves in the spinal cord itself are severed. Both of these operations prevent pain signals from reaching the brain. Pain relief is usually immediate and may last for months. Depending on which nerves are involved in the operation, a variety of side effects can accompany it, ranging from paralysis to numbness and incontinence. Some men in the last stage of their illnesses say these side effects are a small price to pay for freedom from pain.

Nonmedical Approaches

While you can't make your pain disappear by ignoring it, you may be able to think, meditate, or relax it away. So-called alternative approaches to pain management, once viewed with great skepticism by the medical establishment, are now widely accepted and employed.

Nonmedical approaches to pain control include:

- relaxation or meditation techniques
- hypnosis
- acupuncture
- biofeedback
- regular exercise
- distracting yourself with work, a hobby, or pleasurable activity
- imagery
- massage

Detailed descriptions of these are beyond the scope of this book. The pamphlet "Questions and Answers about Pain Control," available free from the Cancer Information Service (800-4-CANCER), explores them a bit more fully. Another good source of information is *You Don't Have to Suffer: A Complete Guide to Relieving Cancer Pain for Patients and Their Families* by Susan Lang and Dr. Richard Patt (New York: Oxford University Press, 1994).

15

Living with Prostate Cancer

The words "You have prostate cancer" trigger a shock that reverberates for years. It ranks right up there with the death of a partner, a parent, or a child. The responses are as different as the sizes, shapes, and personalities of the men who get this disease. Some deal with it as they would a difficult problem at work—attack it logically, identify a solution, carry it out, and then move on to the next problem. Some try to deny the problem and bury its memory as soon as they can. Some men go into emotional shock and turn to a partner, child, or friend to make all the necessary decisions. Some get depressed while others get energized; some become bitter, others more open and accepting. Don't worry about finding the right way to cope. There isn't one—you do what you can to get through. Just getting through would be tough enough if prostate cancer were the kind of disease a man recovered from, like tuberculosis or a bad gallbladder. It's actually more like heart disease or diabetes, something that is with you for years. It is almost impossible to say how much time must elapse before a man can say he is "cured" of prostate cancer—men who have undergone a prostatectomy or radiation therapy for a small, confined tumor can find out ten years later that some cells had escaped the gland before treatment and are now growing in the bones or lymph nodes. Nor is the diagnosis of advanced prostate cancer an immediate death sentence—men with advanced prostate cancer can live for years with their cancer kept in check by hormone therapy.

Everyone diagnosed with prostate cancer—early or advanced, cured or not cured—becomes a survivor, at least for a while. "Survival, in fact, begins at the point of diagnosis, because that is the time when patients are forced to confront their own mortality and begin to make adjustments that will be part of their immediate and, to some extent, long-term future," writes Dr. Fitzhugh Mullan in a moving personal essay about his own battle with cancer.[1] He describes what he calls the seasons of survival for people with cancer. Unfortunately, there's relatively little formal help for men struggling with the problems they face while living through these seasons. "It is as if we have invented sophisticated techniques to save people from drowning, but once they have been pulled from the water, we leave them on the dock to cough and splutter on their own in the belief that we have done all that we can," Mullan writes.

[1] F. Mullan, "Seasons of Survival: Reflections of a Physician with Cancer," *New England Journal of Medicine* 313, (July 25, 1985): 270–273. See also Fitzhugh Mullan and Barbara Hoffman, eds., *Charting the Journey: An Almanac of Practical Resources for Cancer Survivors* (New York: Consumer Reports Books, 1990).

This chapter can't offer you the "postresuscitation" help that Mullan seeks. Nor is it a detailed road map to guide you through the foreign country of prostate cancer. It's more like a compass from a box of Cracker Jack—it points you in the right general direction and, with some work on your part, will get you where you want to go. (See Resources for more detailed publications on coping with cancer.) The sections that follow briefly describe what you might expect to face during the different phases of prostate cancer, each with its own distinct set of problems and adaptations:

- The shock of diagnosis
- Deciding what to do
- Treatment and recovery
- Beyond treatment—living with prostate cancer

This chapter concludes with sections on returning to work during or after treatment for prostate cancer, and paying for your medical care.

Diagnosis

A Thunderbolt from the Blue

Many cancers give vague hints of their presence long before they are ever diagnosed—the hacking cough that precedes lung cancer or the headaches and disorientation that accompany a brain tumor. In a way, these symptoms give one some warning and perhaps a small head start on what lies ahead. With prostate cancer, few men get such signals. The diagnosis usually appears like the proverbial thunderbolt from out of the blue, suddenly striking when a physician feels a hard lump on the prostate or a PSA test comes back well above normal. Glenn, the founder of a small biotechnology company, recalls that he was "in the pink of health" when he learned he had prostate cancer during a routine physical exam just before his sixtieth birthday. "I was looking forward to another five or ten years of work, was playing lots of tennis in the summer and squash during the winter and generally felt fine. I wouldn't believe my doctor when he told me I had prostate cancer. I kept asking, 'How can I have cancer when I feel so good?' "

As the PSA becomes a standard test for men over age fifty, such unexpected diagnoses are now the rule. While the PSA detects tumors at an earlier, potentially more curable stage, it also bursts into a man's life and delivers unexpected bad news. One minute you're relatively healthy with the usual aches and pains of middle age, the next you're a cancer victim facing major therapy. "I just wasn't prepared for anything like this," says sixty-three-year-old Bud. "I made it through Korea without a scratch, never missed a day of work, my heart's in great shape, and I never worry about my bladder like some of my buddies. It just didn't seem right I could feel this good and still need surgery that would lay me up for a few weeks."

While there's never a good time to get cancer, prostate cancer comes at a particularly bad time. It often hits right around retirement, a very vulnerable period when men can lose the structure for their days and weeks, their work friends, and sometimes the defining center of their lives. Prostate cancer often rudely shatters long-relished plans for retirement—spending comfortable, pressure-free time with family or friends, travel, new hobbies, perhaps a move to a city with a warmer climate and slower lifestyle. For some men, prostate cancer further complicates taking care of an ailing partner. It may come on the heels of other health problems such as heart disease, adult-onset diabetes, or early Alzheimer's disease, adding to the sense that things are falling apart and making recovery from treatment more difficult. And finally, prostate cancer often appears just as friends and acquaintances begin passing away, further emphasizing one's mortality.

Whom to Tell

Many men play the prostate cancer card close to the chest, partly because of the fear and misunderstanding still linked to cancer, partly because the prostate's sexual connotation makes people uncomfortable, and partly out of "consideration" for others. Seventy-six-year-old Joseph never told his wife or children about his prostate cancer, and managed to have daily radiation treatments on the sly. "I didn't want to worry them," said the former college professor. But he acknowledged the danger in this approach. "There would have been hell to pay if they ever found out. I know my wife would have been hurt to the core, but I think she would have been frantic with worry if I had told her." There's little question that Joseph's wife would have worried about her husband's health and their future together; that's natural and healthy. But along with that worrying would have come the love and support he definitely could have used during this difficult time.

Most men *do* share their diagnosis with family members. Many take an important step further and involve their partner in making decisions about treatment. After all, she or he shares your life and your future, and treatment will certainly affect both. A partner's love, support, and care can often make this rough period easier, almost normal. Children, too, can provide key help and support. And it probably takes more effort to keep your illness from them. Even young children and grandchildren can grasp the concept that a father or grandfather needs some medical care and some extra special attention for a while. And the pleasure of doing normal things with young ones can offer its own brand of revitalizing therapy.

Be prepared, though, for your children to shy away from one subject related to prostate cancer. Many children don't want to think of their parents as sexually active adults and may turn squeamish—or tune you out altogether—when the issues of impotence or sex come up. Your illness may also raise their own fears about sickness and death.

What about friends, coworkers, and employers? That depends on how comfortable you feel talking about yourself and how well you accept expressions of sorrow and support. You aren't obliged to tell anyone, and it's really no one's business. Share your news only if you want to. If you're working, you'll probably have to tell someone before you begin treatment, otherwise it might be awfully difficult to explain away a several-week absence or thirty-five consecutive days of long lunches or leaving early. (Don't keep quiet about your diagnosis because you fear you may lose your job. Several laws prevent such discrimination. See page 318.)

No matter how gently and kindly you tell others about your cancer, the revelation is bound to make waves you didn't expect. It can strengthen a marriage or widen the cracks that already exist. It can draw children or friends closer, or make them feel guilty about all the things they haven't said or done over the years. It can also make people stay away just when you need them the most. "My best friend never called me once after I told him about my cancer, not when I was in the hospital and not when I was recovering at home," says seventy-one-year-old Barry, a former policeman. "We were never great talkers, but I expected at least a visit or two." After a few months Barry called his friend and they started getting together again. "He finally told me he never knew what to say, and didn't want to talk to me about dying."

If a trusted friend, or even a family member, drops out of the picture during your treatment and recovery, you may have to make the first move. Sometimes just a phone call to tell them you are doing fine and would like to see them is enough to turn things around.

Making Your Decision

A suspicious prostate nodule or an elevated PSA usually sparks a dizzying round of tests—a biopsy, more blood tests, possibly a bone scan. A visit to a urologist or radiation oncologist for a second opinion may leave your head swirling with all the information you receive. (It's sometimes hard to absorb everything during these brief consultations. Don't hesitate to bring along an advocate or interpreter such as a partner or a friend.) You'll probably feel a sense of urgency to complete these tests and appointments as quickly as possible. That's natural, and all for the best. But don't worry if you can't get everything done right away. Prostate cancer rarely spreads like wildfire, so taking two or four weeks isn't going to damage your chances for successful treatment. In fact, taking the time to make a good decision will considerably improve your attitude, outlook, and posttreatment life.

When faced with a life-changing disease like prostate

cancer, it would be great to have a Marcus Welby, M.D., make the necessary decisions for you. But that brand of paternalistic advice has fallen out of favor. Physicians aren't abdicating their responsibility. Instead, they are following healthy trends in medical wisdom and consumer attitudes which suggest that patients should play a role in choosing their own treatment. For several years, women have had to make tough choices regarding breast cancer—whether or not to have a mammogram before age fifty, whether to choose a mastectomy or a lumpectomy for a localized breast tumor, whether to have a breast reconstructed right away, several months later, or not at all. While some women find this emphasis on participation disconcerting, a growing number appreciate having an important say in their treatment. Men now face similar kinds of choices when it comes to prostate cancer.

Your physician really can't make these kinds of decisions for you. "What is right for one patient isn't right for another," says MGH urologist Alex Althausen. "Personal preferences and desires play a huge role in choosing one prostate cancer treatment from several options. Some men can't bear the thought of having cancer inside them, others want to do everything possible to preserve their sex life. As a physician, I can't know what's important to an individual and make the 'right' decision—a man must do that for himself."

Actually, there probably isn't just one treatment that might be right for you. Prostate cancer isn't a one-answer puzzle you have to solve correctly or face the consequences. What you want to do is make a decision that feels right today and will still feel right in six months or six years. Making a good decision doesn't guarantee you success—no treatment does—but it will give you peace of mind and help reduce some of the stress associated with treatment and recovery.

If there were only one treatment for prostate cancer, or if the different treatments had precisely the same side effects, then dealing with this disease would be far simpler than it is. But there are several options for early-stage tumors and several more for advanced tumors; side effects differ from one to the next. Although Chapter 7 describes the decision-making process in greater detail, it doesn't provide a simple algorithm. You can't just plug in your numbers and come out with an answer that's right for you. Instead, you have to become an instant expert in the ever-changing field of prostate cancer and make an expert's decision. That's a tall order, even for a medical professional like seventy-four-year-old Peter, a retired cardiologist. "After plowing through the medical literature, I still wasn't sure I could identify the best treatment for me. That surprised me, because I've been reading about controversies in medicine for forty years. Maybe it's different when you're the one who is going to have to undergo the treatment and suffer any side effects."

Fortunately, you needn't make this decision on your own. Family members and friends can help you do some research on this disease. An even more valuable resource are men who have been down this road before you. Since 1990, more than half a million men have been diagnosed with prostate cancer. Many of them are still alive, and many are eager to share what they've learned and experienced. Don't be bashful about asking for help. You've probably turned to strangers for advice on getting a mortgage or investing money. This is no different, except the stakes are higher and more personal. A growing number of men who have struggled with prostate cancer have become lay experts who are only too happy to help someone else navigate this mine field. You can return the favor in a year or two by helping someone else who has just learned the bad news.

It is not hard to find a fellow member of the prostate-cancer club. Ask your physician if he or she can refer you to a former patient who might be helpful. Call your local hospitals to see if they sponsor any prostate-cancer support groups. Or call one of the national organizations listed in the Resources section.

Don't agree to any treatment before you are ready and feel comfortable with your decision. If it takes you three or four weeks, that's great. On the other hand, don't let caution and the desire to get enough information turn into procrastination. You don't need to consult every specialist in town or ponder your decision for months. Getting a second opinion certainly makes sense. If it yields a recommendation different from the first, a third opinion might be in order. Fourth, fifth, and sixth opinions aren't going to tell you much more, and may even make your decision more difficult. Say you consult the six top prostate cancer specialists in your area. Three recommend a prostatectomy, two say that radiation therapy would be best, and one suggests watchful waiting. You really don't know much more than you did before you started, especially if you liked or trusted all six. If you didn't, you may be inclined to base your choice on the personality of one physician, which might not be the best selection criterion.

Waiting too long to begin treatment can sometimes tip the balance from a potentially curable, localized tumor to an ultimately incurable one that has spread beyond the gland. If you haven't made a decision in a month because you really can't, you may want to talk with a social worker or counselor to help you sort things out.

Treatment and Recovery

Having selected a treatment other than watchful waiting, you'll probably want to get on with it. There's a sense of purpose, a desire to get the worst behind you and get back to your normal life. You'll probably be caught up in all the activity. Daily visits for radiation therapy give your days a clear focus, a feeling of doing something about your cancer. At the same time they make life awfully hectic, especially if you are working and have to sandwich them into your daily routine. Organizing your life around radiation therapy requires some help from family members, coworkers, neighbors, friends. It also means a substantial change in diet if you want to avoid the rectal burning that can accompany radiation. There's no participation in surgery, you are out cold for that. Your involvement comes later, when you focus on the little steps toward recovery—your first solid food, your first walk around the hospital floor, your first bowel movement, going home, doing Kegel exercises, eventually having your catheter removed. Hormone therapy is generally the simplest of the three active treatment options, no matter which method you choose. An orchiectomy is over in a few hours, you're back at home that evening and back to your old routines within a week. Drug therapy usually involves a visit to your physician once a month for an injection of an LHRH agonist such as leuprolide (Lupron). Combined hormone therapy makes life a bit more complicated since it means taking antiandrogen pills every day.

This period of treatment and early recovery can be fraught with emotional turmoil. You'll probably feel vulnerable, even helpless at times. Some men can handle this and graciously accept ministrations from loved ones and friends. Others get angry that they can't fend for themselves. Loved ones can easily misinterpret both the anger and the refusals and think they are doing something wrong. It's difficult to watch someone you love hurt and not be able to help. So do your loved ones a favor—be gracious and let them take care of you.

Throughout the treatment and recovery period, support from family and friends is important. It may be a pot of chicken soup or a good book, a couple hours a week spent mowing your lawn, or daily visits to chat and watch a ballgame on television. Curiously, some of the people who come through for you during this period may not be the ones you had been counting on. Close friends sometimes wait for a signal from you that you are ready for company, not wanting to intrude on your privacy or time with your family. And even though you are the one with cancer, you may end up consoling and reassuring others. "One thing I never, ever could have guessed was how much I was going to have to help other people deal with my cancer," says Barry. "I mean, I sort of got used to the idea that someday I'll probably die from it. But I had to continually help other people deal with it, even my kids and grandkids. That took a lot of energy."

A growing body of research suggests that you may be able to improve the healing power of drugs, surgery, or radiation—or at least improve your quality of life—by tending to your emotions and the rest of your body. All treatments for prostate cancer are what physicians euphemistically call "insults" to the body. Surgery cuts skin, muscles, and blood vessels; radiation kills healthy cells around the prostate; and testosterone-reducing hormone therapy halts the supply of a compound that muscles and other tissues use for growth. All of these treatments can tire you out, weaken your muscles, and depress your immune system. A healthy diet and regular exercise can offset these "insults." Eating right gives you the energy you need each day to maintain your normal health and counteract the negative effects of treatment. A diet that contains plenty of fruits and vegetables delivers an ample daily dose of compounds that fight cancer and bolster the immune system. Exercise lets you regain muscle tone and it, too, can help keep your immune system in shape. It's also a great way of relieving stress.

Reducing stress *may* give you a better shot at beating cancer or living longer with it. Such an idea was once the province of fringe physicians and new-age healers. Now it is gradually becoming part of more mainstream medicine, supported by institutions like the National Institutes of Health's Office of Alternative Medicine, and Harvard Medical School's affiliation with the Mind-Body Institute in Boston. The first rigorously scientific hint that the mind or emotions could play a role in fighting cancer came in 1989 from a ten-year study of women with metastatic breast cancer. Those who participated in a support group during and after treatment and got lessons in self-hypnosis to control pain had twice the survival time of women who received only standard medical therapy. Since then, similar studies have bolstered the concept that the mind can have a direct impact on health and survival with cancer and other diseases. Even though no one knows how or why this works, the message is clear—you may be able to do things for your mind and body that enhance what your treatments can do for your cancer. Best of all, stress reduction or a support group can't hurt—even if they do nothing for one's cancer, they can improve how you feel today and perhaps how you view the future.

One small caution is in order here. While there is no question that you can play an important role in fighting your prostate cancer, the outcome isn't completely up to you. Even men who adopt the healthiest diets, who continue to exercise, who become stress free and think only positive thoughts about the future can have their cancer recur or progress.

Beyond Treatment

"You don't ever totally recover from prostate cancer," says Eli, a seventy-six-year-old baker who underwent a prostatectomy almost ten years ago. "My body is fine, if you forget about the arthritis and a bad hip, but sometimes I still worry that the cancer is going to come back."

Eli makes an excellent point. Treatment, no matter how wonderfully it went, doesn't guarantee you a cure. And since prostate cancer cells grow so slowly, a tiny pocket of cells that had escaped the gland before an operation or radiotherapy may take ten to fifteen years to reappear as a tumor in the lungs, lymph nodes, or bones. Like an unpleasant mother-in-law or an obnoxious neighbor, you'll have to learn to live with the specter of prostate cancer for years. On a purely practical level, this means you should have a checkup at least once a year, complete with rectal exam and PSA test. If some tumor cells have survived and begin to grow, the PSA level will eventually begin climbing.

In a sense, every man diagnosed with prostate cancer ends up following a course of watchful waiting no matter what treatment he has chosen. You sweat every backache, unexplained pelvic pain, shortness of breath, or dribble of urine, and wonder if it is due to a recurrence. For those who have had a prostatectomy or radiation therapy, this worry generally fades over the years. But for those who opted for watchful waiting or who are on hormone therapy, watchfulness and mistrust intensify with time. This medical sword of Damocles prompts quite different responses from men:

"I kind of held back for a few years, waiting for the other shoe to drop before getting back to my old life," says Eli.

Mike, a seventy-three-year-old former draftsman, did just the opposite. "I didn't know how much time I had left and figured I didn't have any time to lose. My wife and I went to Ireland for six months, something we had talked about for years. Then we traveled back and forth across the U.S. Looking back, it was awfully hectic, but I felt like I had to cram in everything I'd ever wanted to do because if I didn't do it now I wasn't going to."

The emotional aftershocks vary. Many men breeze through diagnosis, treatment, and recovery and pick up where they left off without missing a beat. Others enter a changed world, a sudden descent from health and self-sufficiency to illness and dependency, physically and emotionally drained by the experience. "From the day we got married in 1937, my Paul always had five projects going around the house and he was always volunteering for this organization or that. After he retired he seemed even busier than ever. But the cancer kind of took the wind out of his sails, and he just wasn't the same afterward," says seventy-nine-year-old Betty.

Perhaps the biggest danger in the six to twelve months after being diagnosed with prostate cancer is depression. It's a common problem, and a sneaky one. It creeps up on you, often disguised as the aftereffects of treatment—you can't fall asleep at night or sleep far too much; your appetite dwindles; you don't get much pleasure out of seeing friends or pursuing old hobbies. Depression isn't anything to be ashamed of. You've been fighting a life-threatening illness, and may be facing life-changing complications. You may have lost some of your normal support networks at home or at work. Or you may be facing the certainty of your own mortality for the first time. Who wouldn't be depressed?

Being down in the dumps for a while is different from depression, a medically recognized problem with some potentially serious consequences. Long-lasting depression appears to interfere with the body's ability to heal or defend itself from infection; it can lead to suicide. Here are some of depression's warning signs:

- A sense of helplessness or despair
- An inability to sleep
- A loss of appetite
- Irritability
- Inability to get pleasure from formerly enjoyable activities

Merely recognizing depression may be enough to make it begin evaporating. Sometimes it disappears all by itself—you wake one morning and really notice a blue sky, your partner's smile, the sound of music. More often than not, though, getting rid of this emotional and physical funk takes some professional help. Talking with a counselor, social worker, or therapist is an excellent start. He or she may recommend a short course of antidepressants to get you over the hump. Another solution may be a prostate-cancer support group. You'll realize you aren't alone and perhaps make some new friends to boot.

For a while, prostate cancer will dominate your life, your thoughts, your moods and emotions. At some point, though, the rest of your life will begin to reassert itself and shove your illness aside. Grandchildren you've neglected, a hobby you've put aside, volunteer work you've stopped, your "old" life will come knocking at your door. You'll answer when you are ready.

Back to Work

As physicians get better and better at detecting prostate cancer, more young men—those under age sixty-five—are diagnosed with this disease each year. They face the special burden of holding on to a job during treatment and recovery, as do the men who continue working after age sixty-five because they want to, or because they need the money. Most merely face the hassle of taking time off for surgery and its recovery period, or finding a way to fit seven or eight weeks of daily radiation treatments into an already hectic daily schedule. A few men, unfortunately, also face employers and coworkers who harbor outdated notions of cancer, or struggle with intractable bureaucracies over benefits and insurance.

You may feel awkward when you return to work after treatment, or keep working when others know you have cancer. Conversations at work often focus on the job or sports or the news and tend to gloss over personal problems such as a rocky marriage, troublesome children, or mounting bills. Add cancer to these taboo subjects. Your coworkers won't want to bring up the subject of prostate cancer for fear of upsetting you, or because they feel they're invading your privacy. Their reticence may also stem from ignorance—a surprising number of people still harbor the totally false notion that everyone diagnosed with cancer has only a few months to live, or that cancer can be contagious. Some may be worried that your illness will jack up everyone's health insurance premiums.

As with virtually every phase of living with cancer, you have to take the initiative. The more open you are about this very common disease, the less your coworkers will studiously avoid the subject. Everyone benefits. "When I had my prostatectomy, I kept pretty quiet about the whole thing," says Bob, a fifty-five-year-old publishing company vice president. "A few months later when I started radiation treatments, I tried to do the same thing. But as I had to let more and more people know, because of rescheduling projects and meetings, it got easier to talk about. And I was floored how kind and thoughtful and supportive people were. It made a big difference."

Respect others' limits, though. Few, if any, of your colleagues want to know the gory details of your prostatectomy, how many pads you go through each day in order to stay dry, or what treatment you're testing to combat impotence.

Workplace conversation isn't the only issue. Managers and coworkers often don't know what to expect from you when you return to work, or while you are undergoing radiation or hormone therapy. They may rearrange your schedule or reduce your responsibilities without first asking if such changes are okay with you. This is generally their way of trying to make things easier for you, often done on the QT because people find it hard to broach the subject of cancer. If this is your colleagues' way of pitching in and supporting you—the same kind of thing you might do for someone else—accept their help and let them know how much you appreciate it. But if their attention or your changed responsibilities make you uncomfortable, speak up. Let your supervisor and coworkers know exactly what you can, and can't, do.

If you find yourself returning to a lower-paying job or one a few notches down in the hierarchy, or believe you are being slowly eased out of the company, raise your concerns with your supervisor or the head of personnel. If you aren't satisfied with the results of your inquiries, keep in mind that several state and federal laws may work in your favor:

- The Americans with Disabilities Act. Passed in 1992, this law protects the rights of people with a handicap or disability. It covers anyone with a major health problem that affects the ability to do everyday activities at home or at work. Cancer falls into this category, at least during the period when it poses a health threat. Businesses with fifteen or more employees are required to make "reasonable accommodation" for someone with a disability or handicap. This includes being flexible about responsibilities or hours so you can get the treatment you need. However, employers don't necessarily have to do this if the accommodation places an undue financial or staffing burden on the company.

- The Family and Medical Leave Act. Any company with fifty or more employees must now let a worker take up to twelve weeks of unpaid leave so he or she can deal with an illness such as cancer; or care for a sick spouse, child, or parent; or care for a new baby or an adopted child. The company must either hold your job open for you or give you an equivalent one when you return. And it must also provide you with full benefits, including health insurance, during the leave.

Cancer survivors sometimes face problems when they look for work or try to change jobs. Prospective employers often ask about past or present illnesses, and job applications generally include questions about your health history. By law, an employer can't pass you over for a job because of your health. In practice, though, it happens all the time.

If you feel you are being discriminated against at work because of your prostate cancer, or are fairly certain a prospective employer didn't hire you because of your medical history, there are several places to turn for help.

• The National Coalition for Cancer Survivorship (see Resources) has been dealing with this issue since its inception. Its pamphlet, "Working It Out: Your Employment Rights As a Cancer Survivor," offers an excellent overview of your rights and how to get help.

• Most states have an office or agency or commission that deals with discrimination issues. If you can burrow your way through the state bureaucracy and find the right office, you will likely get detailed, helpful information.

• The federal Equal Opportunity Employment Commission can also provide you with information about your workplace rights as a cancer survivor. The EEOC's Public Information System, 800-669-4000, can direct you to the agency in your state that handles these issues. It also has a variety of publications on your rights in the workplace. You can get a list by calling 800-669-EEOC.

Paying for Treatment

In addition to the physical and emotional tolls that prostate cancer exacts, men often pay a financial price as well. Lost wages can shrink a bank account as surely as the hefty cost of treatment. The escalating costs of modern medicine haven't bypassed prostate cancer. Except for watchful waiting, treatment can easily cost more than $10,000.

Diagnostic tests and the so-called standard treatments—prostatectomy, radiation therapy, orchiectomy, hormone therapy, and lymph-node sampling—are usually covered by general medical insurance such as Blue Cross, an HMO, or Medicare. Insurance that pays for complete prostate care, from diagnostic PSA to therapy and follow-up, provides some peace of mind during an already trying time. Scrambling for the money to pay for a prostatectomy or radiation or the drugs needed for hormone therapy adds an unnecessary and stressful burden. If cancer puts you in a financial bind, talk with your physician. He or she knows how the system works and may be able to point out some options you would have overlooked.

Finding Funds

If you are working full-time, odds are you have medical insurance through your employer. Your company's benefits expert can tell you exactly what your insurance will cover. If you are sixty-five or older you qualify for Medicare, the federal medical insurance program administered through the Social Security Administration. It pays for standard diagnostic tests and treatment strategies, including those for incontinence and impotence that result from cancer therapy. It may not, however, cover the cost of drugs needed for hormone therapy or chemotherapy. You can buy extra "Medigap" insurance that will cover prescription drugs, home care, and other medical necessities.

If you have served in the armed forces, see if you qualify for cancer treatment at a nearby Veterans Affairs medical center. For questions about veterans' benefits, call 800-827-1000.

The American Cancer Society (800-ACS-2345) also provides information about funding cancer treatment. Some local ACS offices can help with transportation to and from your home and medical center, or may be able to help you pay for drugs or necessary medical devices.

Some pharmaceutical companies operate programs that help cancer patients pay for expensive drugs. Your physician or urologist should know of any that apply to prostate-cancer treatment.

A federal program called Hill-Burton requires hospitals that receive construction funds from the federal government to offer care for people who can't afford to pay for their hospitalization. To find out if you are eligible, or for a list of Hill-Burton hospitals in your area, call 800-638-0742.

Dealing with Insurers

When it comes to a major illness such as prostate cancer, merely *having* insurance isn't always enough. You must make it work for you, something that takes time, patience, organization, and some moxie. In addition to coping with your cancer and treatment, you may have to become an accountant to make sure your insurance pays for everything it should. So you don't have to.

Keep accurate records of the visits you make to your

physician and any specialists, as well as the tests and procedures you undergo. Make a special folder, or set aside a drawer for the bills you get—it's easier to deal with them when they are all in one place. When you get a bill, hang on to the original and send only copies to your insurers. Finally, don't let bills pile up for several months. A mountain of unpaid bills can overwhelm and disappoint you. On a more practical level, some insurance companies have a one-year statute of limitations.

Be prepared for rejection. It's not uncommon for an insurer to return a claim unpaid, or pay only a fraction of the bill for a test or medical procedure. If this happens, try resubmitting the claim. Odds are it will be reviewed by a different claims adjuster who might allow it. If that doesn't work, an invaluable pamphlet called "What Cancer Survivors Need to Know About Health Insurance," published by the National Coalition for Cancer Survivorship, suggests attaching a note to the rejected claim saying "Please review this claim." And if that doesn't work, submit the claim yet again with a note asking that it be reviewed by "peer review physicians."

Treatments considered experimental, investigational, or alternative immediately raise red flags for insurers. Most don't readily cover anything outside of the medical mainstream. Often excluded are cryosurgery, radioactive seed implants, some forms of hormone therapy or chemotherapy, and alternative therapies such as creative visualization, antineoplastons, or herbal treatments. But it never hurts to try. You and your physician may be able to marshal enough evidence to persuade an insurer to cover the cost. That means convincing the insurer that the therapy is no longer considered experimental, or that it benefits a defined group of people and you fall into that group. The

Association of Community Cancer Centers publishes a booklet called "Cancer Treatments Your Insurance Should Cover" that should help you figure out what's considered standard therapy.

For more information about paying for prostate cancer or dealing with insurers, you can turn to several excellent resources. The prostate-cancer support and lobbying group called PAACT (Patient Advocates for Advanced Cancer Treatments) has become quite involved in insurance issues concerning prostate cancer. As mentioned above, the National Coalition for Cancer Survivorship has also assembled a raft of helpful information. Your state department of insurance can send you information on current state laws and your insurance rights.

Resources

We have tried to make this book a comprehensive guide to prostate disease. But you may still want to gather more information, or connect with other men who are dealing with prostate disease. This section will point you to organizations, books, and electronic resources that we think you might find helpful. One caution about what you may encounter on the Internet: Online services or bulletin boards offer a fast, easy way to find information. Unfortunately, it is tough to tell whether it's good information or nonsense, since anyone can sound like an expert and you never really know who you are "talking" to. So take what you find with a grain of salt, and check it out with a physician or other clinician whose opinion you respect.

Any Prostate Disease

American Foundation for Urologic Disease
300 W. Pratt St.
Baltimore, MD 21201
800-242-2383

This foundation funds research on all urologic diseases, and serves as an information clearinghouse for men with prostatitis, BPH, and prostate cancer.

National Kidney and Urologic Diseases Information
Clearinghouse
Box NKUDIC
Bethesda, MD 20892
301-654-4415

Part of the National Institutes of Health, this clearinghouse provides information on all prostate diseases. For the price of a long-distance phone call, a research specialist will track down pamphlets, research papers, and other published information.

Prostatitis

The Prostatitis Foundation
2029 Ireland Grove Road
Bloomington, IL 61704
309-664-6222

Started in June 1995, this nonprofit, volunteer-run organization helps men with prostatitis find the most appropriate treatment for their ailment and share their experiences with fellow prostatitis sufferers via a phone bank. The Prostate Foundation also has a useful World Wide Web page that can point you to other prostate resources on the Internet:
    <http://www.prostate.org>

A lively newsgroup on the Internet also offers a forum for commiseration and the exchange of ideas:

  <sci.med.prostate.prostatitis>

Benign Prostatic Hyperplasia

For a free copy of the Agency for Health Care Policy Research's guidelines on BPH, call or write:

AHCPR Publications Clearinghouse
PO Box 8547
Silver Spring, MD 20907
800-358-9295
Ask for *Benign Prostatic Hyperplasia: Diagnosis and Treatment.*

An Internet discussion group created in October 1995 deals specifically with benign prostatic hyperplasia:

  <sci.med.prostate.bph>

Prostate Cancer

General Information

Prostate Cancer Support Network
300 W. Pratt, Suite 401
Baltimore, MD 21201
800-828-7866

The Prostate Cancer Support Network provides up-to-date information about prostate diseases. Equally important, it can point you to an Us-Too support group in your area.

American Cancer Society
(chapters in all states)
800-ACS-2345

The American Cancer Society offers general information on cancer, cancer treatment, and coping with cancer, as well as referrals to local meetings of Man to Man. Some local chapters offer help with transportation to and from treatment centers.

Cancer Information Service
800-4-CANCER

This free service, sponsored by the National Cancer Institute, provides specific, detailed information about all kinds of cancer and cancer treatment. Tell the research assistant as much as you can about your cancer, and he or she will search through a huge national database and send you the most up-to-date information about treatments, including a list of cancer centers near you.

National Coalition for Cancer Survivorship
1010 Wayne Ave., 5th floor
Silver Spring, MD 20910
301-650-8868

Survivorship begins the moment you are diagnosed with cancer. This organization offers detailed information to help you live and cope with cancer. Workplace and discrimination issues are a specialty.

Cancer Care Counseling Line
1180 Avenue of the Americas
New York, NY 10036
800-813-HOPE

Sponsored by Cancer Care, a national agency that provides psychological and social support for people with cancer and their families. A call to the toll-free number will connect you with a social worker who can offer emotional support or invaluable guidance about doctor-patient communication, second opinions, and coping with cancer, as well as direct you to local organizations that may be able to provide transportation, home care, or assistance with pain management.

Support Groups

Not only do the groups listed below offer reassurance and emotional support, but they can also offer valuable education and information that's often unavailable from your physician.

Us-Too
930 N. York Road, Suite 50
Hinsdale, IL 60521-2993
800-808-7866

This national organization, modeled after the highly successful Y-ME for women with breast cancer, organizes support groups across the country.

Man-to-Man
c/o American Cancer Society
800-ACS-2345

Another support group network with chapters from coast to coast.

Patient Advocates for Advanced Cancer Treatments
1143 Parmelee Ave., NW
Grand Rapids, MI 49504
616-453-1477

An information and lobbying group dedicated to improving treatment for early- and late-stage prostate cancer. While much of the information that PAACT makes available is very useful, the organization tends to promote new and as-yet-unproven treatments before their time.

Prostate Cancer Online

A rapidly expanding array of prostate cancer resources and sites are scattered across the Internet and the World Wide Web. They range from thoughtful, compassionate discussions by and about men with prostate cancer to shameless hucksters trying to sell the equivalent of modern-day snake oil.

One of the best sites is the prostate cancer discussion group on Prodigy. Jump to the MEDICAL BB, select the CANCER topic, then select the PROSTATE CANCER library. CompuServe and America Online also have lively discussion groups.

For the Internet savvy, a prostate cancer Usenet group serves up daily discussions about treatments for prostate cancer and new research on this disease. Men frequently go online to ask advice about a rising PSA or suitable treatment options:

<sci.med.prostate.cancer>

Two World Wide Web pages, both of which contain helpful links to other Web sites, can get you started surfing the Internet for prostate resources:

<http://www.comed.com/prostate>
<http://oncolink.upenn.edu/disease/prostate/index.html>

Incontinence and Impotence

Help for Incontinent People
PO Box 544
Union, SC 29379
800-BLADDER

For straight talk on living with incontinence and information on ways to beat it.

Resolve, Inc.
1310 Broadway
Somerville, MA 02144-1731
617-623-0744

Resolve helps people with infertility problems. The organization
offers information on medical therapies as well as adoption. It
can most likely refer you to a medical specialist or sperm bank
in your area.

Impotence Information Center
11001 Bren Road East
Minnetonka, MN 55343
800-843-4315
(612-933-4666 in Minnesota)

Offers educational brochures that describe a variety of treatments for impotence.

Impotents Anonymous (IA)
119 South Ruth Street
Maryville, TN 37803-5746
(615) 983-6064

Impotents Anonymous (IA) is part of the nonprofit Impotence
Institute of America, Inc. which was established in 1983. It will
provide you with a list of professionals who deal with impotence as well as information on joining or starting an IA group.

American Association of Sex Educators, Counselors, and
Therapists
435 N. Michigan Ave., Suite 1717
Chicago, IL 60611
312-644-0828

This professional organization can direct you to a certified
counselor or therapist near your city.

Alternative Therapies

Information on alternative therapies for prostate cancer abounds in tabloids like *East West* or virtually any New Age healing magazine. Please keep in mind that few alternative therapies have been rigorously tested. One or two testimonials do not prove that a therapy has any curative power. An excellent resource on alternative therapies is the book *Choices in Healing: Integrating the Best of Conventional and Complementary Approaches to Cancer.* (Cambridge, Mass.: MIT Press, 1994). Author Michael Lerner, whose father, the noted essayist Max Lerner, battled prostate cancer, has written a thoughtful guide to the full spectrum of alternative therapy, from diets to visualization.

Pain

For a free copy of the Agency for Health Care Policy Research's guidelines on managing cancer pain, call or write:
AHCPR Publications Clearinghouse
PO Box 8547
Silver Spring, MD 20907
800-358-9295
Ask for *Management of Cancer Pain.*

Wisconsin Cancer Pain Initiative
1300 University Ave.
Madison, WI 53706
608-262-0978

Educational pamphlets and videotapes about pain control, as well as information about pain initiatives in other states

National Chronic Pain Outreach Association
7979 Old Georgetown Road, Suite 100
Bethesda, MD 20814
301-652-4948

Disseminates information on chronic pain and its management. The association acts as a clearinghouse of information for those in pain, their families, and health care professionals. It can also make referrals to pain specialists and local chronic pain support groups.

A comprehensive guide on the subject of cancer pain is the book *You Don't Have to Suffer: A Complete Guide to Relieving Cancer Pain for Patients and Their Families* (New York: Oxford University Press, 1994) by Susan Lang and Richard Pratt.

Paying for Prostate Cancer

National Coalition for Cancer Survivorship
1010 Wayne Ave., 5th floor
Silver Spring, MD 20910
301-650-8868

The National Coalition for Cancer Survivorship has excellent brochures that deal with discrimination against cancer survivors, and getting the most out of your insurance company.

Association of Community Cancer Centers
11600 Nebel St., Suite 201
Rockville, MD 20852
301-984-9496

Write for a helpful pamphlet called ``Cancer Treatments Your Insurance Should Cover.''

Medicare Telephone Hotline
800-638-6833

For information on Medicare and Medigap insurance and policies.

National Hospice Organization
1901 N. Moore St., Suite 901
Arlington, VA 22209
800-658-8898

Hospice care is a wonderful alternative to hospitalization for people in the last stage of a terminal illness. The National Hospice Organization provides information on the different kinds of hospice care available, and can refer you to local resources.

Depression Awareness, Recognition and Treatment Program
National Institute of Mental Health
5600 Fishers Lane, Room 15C-05
Rockville, MD 20857
800-421-4211

For information on recognizing the signs of clinical depression, and what to do about it.

Index

About the Authors

W. SCOTT McDOUGAL, M.D., is professor of surgery at Harvard Medical School and chief of urology at Massachusetts General Hospital. An international authority on urology, he is a trustee of the American Board of Urology and former chairman of the American Foundation for Urologic Disease's Research Committee. He lives with his wife in Manchester, Massachusetts.

P. J. SKERRETT is executive editor of *Clinical Care for Prostatic Diseases* and senior writer for *HealthNews,* two newsletters from the publishers of the *New England Journal of Medicine.* He also contributes regularly to *American Health, Popular Science,* and *Technology Review.* He lives with his family in Boston.